Classical Neurotransmitters and Neuropeptides Involved in Schizoaffective Disorder
Focus on Prophylactic Medication

Authored By

Felix-Martin Werner

Euro Akademie Pößneck
Higher Vocational School for Elderly Care and Occupational Therapy
Carl-Gustav-Vogel-Str. 13
07381 Pößneck
Germany

&

Rafael Coveñas

University of Salamanca
Institute of Neurosciences of Castilla y León (INCYL)
Laboratory of Neuroanatomy of the Peptidergic Systems (Lab.14)
c/Pintor Fernando Gallego, 1
37007-Salamanca, Spain

DEDICATION

I dedicate this eBook to my colleagues and friends Günter Brandler, Gera und Jürgen Werner, Mechernich.

Felix-Martin Werner

I dedicate this eBook to my wife Mercedes and to my children Rafael and María

Rafael Coveñas

CONTENTS

FOREWORD

It is an honor for me to write the foreword for the e-book "Classical neurotransmitters and neuropeptides involved in schizoaffective disorder: focus on prophylactic medication" by Dr. Felix-Martin Werner and Dr. Rafael Coveñas. Almost every productive and fantastic work in medicine is the result of expertise in different fields coming together and work towards the best interest of the patients and the scientific/academic community in particular and the mankind in general.

Psychiatric disorders in human make up a large group of mental diseases with a range of sign and symptoms that are caused by genetic problems and biological factors, stress, brain trauma, toxic substances and infections particularly during pregnancy that may affect the embryo, cancers, drug abuse and a history of abuse among many other causes that all may interfere with the normal brain performance by changing the structure and function of the different parts of the nervous system.

Several of these conditions lead to mental disorders due to an imbalance in the metabolism of neurotransmitters and neuromodulators among them, the neuropeptides. More information about mental disorders can be found elsewhere: http://psychcentral.com/disorders/ and https://www.nlm.nih.gov/medlineplus/mentaldisorders.html.

Schizoaffective disorder is believed to be due to continuous psychotic behaviours accompanied by intermittent mood episodes such as major depressive and/or manic episodes. Several neurotransmitters have been implicated in schizophrenia and mood disorders. These include the dopamine in the case of schizophrenia and serotonin, dopamine and adrenaline among others in mood disorders. The hypothalamic neurohormonal pathway and a number of neuropeptides have also been implicated in schizoaffective disorder. Treatment with antipsychotic drugs, mood stabilizers and antidepressant medications is aimed to normalize the neurotransmitter(s) level while talk and group therapies, social support and work training aim to improve patients' daily functions and social behaviour through other methods. There are still many unknowns and facts to learn in this field as sign and symptoms and the treatment outcome may differ from patient to patient.

The current book is a very well written and easy to understand comprehensive text of schizoaffective disorder dissecting the brain and other regions involved in the disease and its pathophysiology, describing the various causes of the disease including the genetic and epigenetics and its current and various modes of treatments and future directions.

The current e-book "Classical neurotransmitters and neuropeptides involved in schizoaffective disorder: focus on prophylactic medication" by Dr. Werner and Dr. Coveñas is a unique collection of practical details and case reports and is a great asset to education, research, and clinical practice of psychiatry and psychology.

Mohtashem Samsam
Burnett School of Biomedical Sciences (BSBS),
College of Medicine, University of Central Florida,
4000 Central Florida Blvd., HPA-II 320
Orlando, FL 32816
USA

PREFACE

Patients with a schizoaffective disorder are met regularly in the psychiatrist's practice and in psychiatric wards. Schizophrenic and affective symptoms show a great variety and the courses of the disease can have different outcomes. For patients' rehabilitation and social integration into the familiar and, in some cases working lives, a prophylactic medication is of great importance. Because we have been working on classical neurotransmitters and neuropeptides involved in schizophrenia and in affective diseases, we describe here the alterations of these neuroactive substances in the brain regions involved in the schizophrenic and affective symptoms. In that way, possibilities of finding new agents acting at specific receptors of classical neurotransmitters and neuropeptides are pointed out. The schizoaffective disorder, which has a prevalance of 0.5% in the population, is undoubtedly an inheritable disease with an environment-gene interaction. Some of the discovered susceptibility genes and the functions of the encoded neuroactive substances involved in the pathophysiology of the disease are pointed out. We have established the relationships between the hypothalamic-adrenal axis and the altered neural networks found in the brain areas involved in schizophrenic and affective symptoms. Because we have published several review articles about neural networks in schizophrenia and major depression, we extended here these neural networks to the brain regions involved in schizophrenic and affective symptoms. An essential chapter has been focused on the prophylactic medication. The different prophylactic medications consider the different forms of the disease. Besides, adverse effects and disease symptoms are mentioned, and the additional pharmacotherapies of these adverse effects and symptoms are mentioned, including the current availabe drugs. Some recently developed antipsychotic drugs such as lurasidone and cariprazine with a different mechanism of action are included as well. Patients' well being is very important. Therefore, it is essential to choose an appropriate prophylactic drug and to support the patients' adherence to the pharmacotherapy through psychoeducation and a social integration. Moreover, this e-book gives a hint to pharmaceutical firms to improve the prophylactic medication by presenting the specific subreceptors involved, on which new pharmacological agents could exert an improved or additional therapeutic effect.

ACKNOWLEDGEMENTS

The authors would like to thank Mr. Nikolas Skinner (University of Salamanca, Spain) for revising the English language.

CONFLICT OF INTEREST

The authors declare that this ebook contents have no conflicts of interest.

Felix-Martin Werner
Euro Akademie Pößneck
Higher Vocational School for Elderly Care and
Occupational Therapy
Carl-Gustav-Vogel-Str. 13
07381 Pößneck
Germany
E-mail: felixm-werner@versanet.de

Rafael Coveñas
University of Salamanca
Institute of Neurosciences of Castilla y León
(INCYL)
Laboratory of Neuroanatomy of the Peptidergic
Systems (Lab.14)
c/ Pintor Fernando Gallego, 1
37007-Salamanca
Spain
E-mail: covenas@usal.es

CHAPTER 1

Classical Neurotransmitters and Neuropeptides Involved in Schizoaffective Disorder: Focus on Prophylactic Medication

INTRODUCTION

Abstract: Schizoaffective disorder has a prevalance of 0.5 %. In this disease, psychotic symptoms are combined with affective, i.e. depressive, manic or bipolar symptoms. The disease is encoded in susceptibility genes, which can be enhanced by stresssful life events or psychotomimitic substances. The neurotransmitter and neuropeptide alterations are described in the involved brain regions in schizophrenic and affective symptoms. In these brain regions, neural networks are described including a multi-neurotransmitter system. The coherence between the hypothalamic-pituitary-adrenal axis and the neurotransmitter alterations will be pointed out. The current pharmacotherapy is reviewed, and some new antipsychotic drugs will be examined critically. The importance of additional sociotherapies and psychoeducaction is underlined, because it enables the schizoaffective patients to be reintegrated into social and perhaps professional lifes.

Keywords: Affective symptom, antipsychotic drug, cognitive symptom, depressive symptom, dopamine, first-episode schizophrenia, gene-environment interaction, hippocampus, manic symptom, mesolimbic system, midbrain, monoamine, negative symptom, neural network, positive symptom, prefrontal cortex, schizoaffective disorder, schizophrenia, serotonin, susceptibility gene,

While schizophrenia, a chronic disabling disorder has a prevalence of 1%, schizoaffective disorder has a prevalence of 0.5%. Schizophrenia, which is associated with positive (paranoia, acoustic hallucinations, illusions), negative (social withdrawal, autism, mutism) and cognitive symptoms, becomes manifest as an acute psychosis with mostly positive symptoms after a prodromal phase of about 7 years [1-3]. Patients suffering from acute psychosis are mostly in their early adolescence years, and men tend to be younger than women when first-episode schizophrenia is diagnosed [4]. When a schizoaffective disorder is diagnosed, positive schizophrenic symptoms are combined with affective symptoms: for example, depressive, manic or bipolar symptoms [5]. An important issue in all this is the reason for the appearance of schizoaffective disorder. In most cases, susceptibility genes have been found. While common susceptibility genes, which encode dopamine hyperactivity through decreased dopamine breakdown or which encode GABA or glutamate hypofunction [4], cause disease

Felix-Martin Werner and Rafael Coveñas

symptoms that can be treated with conventional antipsychotic drugs, rare genes also have an important effect [4]. The severity of acute psychosis is enhanced by environmental factors (*e.g.*, childhood trauma) or the use of psychotomimetic substances (*e.g.*, cannabinoid exposure) [6], since there are gene-environment interactions [4]. In acute psychosis, alterations in neurotransmitters, for example dopamine and serotonin hyperactivity, occur in the mesolimbic system, the hippocampus and the prefrontal cortex. Stressful life events can enhance neurotransmitter alterations in these brain regions. Dopamine hyperactivity is correlated with a dysfunction of the hypothalamic-pituitary-adrenal (HPA) axis and with increased cortisol levels. Consequently, alterations in cortisol levels and increased levels of corticotropin-releasing hormone (CRH) are correlated with increased dopamine levels in the mesolimbic system and hippocampus [4]. This coherence is discussed below, where the neural networks in the brain regions involved in schizophrenia are described. In most schizophrenic or schizoaffective patients, increased cortisol levels are found and the dexamethasone stress test reveals the non-suppression of cortisol levels. Dysfunction of the HPA axis is correlated with psychotic symptoms and cognitive deficits [4]. Moreover, HPA axis dysfunction is associated with patients' vulnerability in stressful situations. In schizoaffective patients, alterations in neurotransmitter and neuropeptide levels can be found in different brain regions [7, 8]. Affective symptoms, for example depressive and manic symptoms, may be associated with a dysfunction of the HPA axis. The correlation between increased CRH levels in the hypothalamus and decreased serotonin levels in the brainstem will be addressed in the chapter about neural networks in the brain regions involved in affective symptoms [7]. In the mesolimbic system and hippocampus, positive schizophrenic symptoms are correlated *via* D_2 and 5-HT_{2A} receptors with dopamine and serotonin hyperactivity [8]. Moreover, in these brain regions a multi-neurotransmitter system has been reported, in which a hypofunction of GABAergic and glutaminergic neurons exerting a presynaptic inhibitory action occurs. In the prefrontal cortex, an antagonistic interaction between M_4 muscarinic cholinergic and D_1 dopaminergic neurons has been described, while agonism at M_4 receptors and a D_1 antagonistic effect exert antipsychotic properties. In the midbrain and hippocampus, the monamines serotonin, noradrenaline and dopamine play an important role in the pathophysiology of depressive and manic symptoms [8]. In the midbrain and hippocampus, a multi-neurotransmitter system will be described, including postsynaptic excitatory neurotransmitters (serotonin, noradrenaline, dopamine, acetylcholine); presynaptic inhibitory neurotransmitters (GABA), and neurotransmitters (glutamate) that exert an excitotoxic and a partly presynaptic inhibitory action [8].

Among the susceptibility genes for schizophrenic symptoms, the common genes encode dopamine hyperactivity through a decreased dopamine breakdown or encode GABA and glutamate hypoactivity [8]. The depressive or manic symptoms are mostly correlated with polymorphisms of the monoamine transporter genes [7]. In this e-book, the relationship between the function of the susceptibility genes and the cellular mechanisms involved will be addressed.

Patients with psychotic symptoms show a worsening of the psychopathology when they are exposed to stressful events or trauma [9]. Patients suffering from acute psychosis should be treated in a psychiatric ward, since it is difficult to reintegrate them into social life and motivate them to return to work [4]. Among the antipsychotic drugs, second-generation antipsychotic drugs (SGAs) are the compounds of choice to treat these patients [10]. Although schizoaffective disorder has a somewhat better outcome than schizophrenia, the number of schizoaffective patients who cannot be reintegrated into social and professional life has not yet been reduced to any meaningful extent [4, 5]. Among the three patients described here in the case reports, two of them are the beneficiaries of a state pension and the other one receives half a pension and performs a part-time work.

Some SGAs such as risperidone, olanzapine, quetiapine, aripiprazole and the most effective SGA, clozapine, will be compared on the basis of their effectiveness [10]. Thus, the antipsychotic and adverse effects of SGAs such as risperidone, which is a D_2 and $5-HT_{2A}$ antagonist and shows high affinity for the D_2 receptor, will be compared with other SGAs, such as quetiapine, which has a D_2 and $5-HT_{2A}$ antagonistic effect and high affinity for the $5-HT_{2A}$ receptor [10]. Clozapine, which has a D_3, D_4 and $5-HT_{2A}$ antagonistic effect, is used in some schizoaffective patients because in spite of its adverse effects (agranulocytosis, neutropenia) it exerts a greater antipsychotic effect than other SGAs. Some promising new SGAs will be discussed and their therapeutic effects will be examined in clinical trials. Examples are lurasidone, asenapine and cariprazine. Lurasidone has a D_2 and $5-HT_{2A}$ antagonistic and a $5-HT_{1A}$ agonistic effect, improving cognitive functions by exerting an additional $5-HT_7$ antagonistic effect. Cariprazine has a good antipsychotic effect *via* a D_2 and D_3 partial agonism, and this has confirmed in clinical trials [10, 11]. Most physicians combine SGAs with mood-stabilizing drugs such as, lithium, topiramate, lamotrigine, valproic acid or carbamazepine [12]. The question arises of whether the combination of SGAs with mood-stabilizing drugs has a better therapeutic effect in comparison with the administration of SGAs alone [12]. The adverse effects of the different antipsychotic and mood-stabilizing drugs will be also compared [13]. Moreover, consideration will be given to the issue of whether sociotherapy, for example a family therapy intervention or integration into a self-help group and psychoeducation, can be helpful in preventing the recurrence of psychotic and affective symptoms. Psychoeducation enables patients to deal with stressful situations and to recognize psychotic or basic symptoms [10].

REFERENCES

[1]   Klosterkötter J. Indicated prevention of schizophrenia. Dtsch Arztebl Int 2008; 105: 532- 9.
[2]   Huber G, Gross G. The concept of basic symptoms in schizophrenic and schizoaffective psychoses. Recent Prog Med 1989; 80: 464-52.
[3]   Werner F-M, Coveñas R. Classical neurotransmitters and neuropeptides involved in schizophrenia: How to choose the appropriate antipsychotic drug? Curr Drug Ther 2013; 8: 132-43.
[4]   Haller SC, Padmanabhan JL, Lizano P, Torous J, Keshavan M. Recent advances in understanding schizophrenia. F1000 Prime Reports 2014; 6: 57.
[5]   Werner F-M, Coveñas R. Treatment of the schizoaffective disorder according to a neuronal network. Klin Neurophysiol 2012, 43:103-4.
[6]   Renard J, Krebs M-O, Le Pen G, Jay TM. Long-term consequences of adolescent cannabinoid exposure in adult psychopathology. Front Neurosci 2014; 8: 361.
[7]   Werner F-M, Coveñas R. Classical neurotransmitters and neuropeptides involved in major depression: a review. Int J Neurosci 2010; 120: 455-70.
[8]   Werner F-M, Coveñas R. Classical neurotransmitters and neuropeptides involved in major depression: a focus on antidepressant drugs. Curr Med Chem 2013; 20:4853-8.
[9]   Ruby E, Polito S, McMahon K, Gorovitz M, Corcoran C, Malaspina D. Pathways associating childhood trauma to the neurobiology of schizophrenia. Front Psychol Behav Sci 2014; 3: 1-17.
[10]   Werner F-M, Coveñas R. Safety of antipsychotic drugs: focus on therapeutic and adverse effects. Exp Opin Drug Saf 2014; 13: 1031-42.
[11]   Calabrese JR, Keck PE Jr., Starace A, *et al.* Efficacy and safety of low- and high-dose cariprazine in acute and mixed mania ssociated with bipolar I disorder: a double-blind, placebo-controlled study. J Clin Psychiatry 2015; 76: 284-92.
[12]   Rajina P. Antiepileptic drugs as mood stabilizers: what did we learn from the epileptology? Ideggyogy Sz 2008; 61: 305-16.
[13]   Ketter TA, Wang PW, Becker OV, Nowakowska C, Yang YS. The diverse roles of anticonvulsants in bipolar disorders. Ann Clin Psychiatry 2003; 15: 95-108.

CHAPTER 2

Forms of Schizoaffective Disorder and Case Reports

Abstract: Here, we describe the forms of schizoaffective disorder with schizophrenic and affective symptoms, for example depressive or manic symptoms or the bipolar form. Prognosis of the schizoaffective disorder is better than that of schizophenia and there are three different outcomes: a schizoaffective psychosis with a total remission, recurrent psychoses with a residual condition and recurrent psychoses with a deficiency condition. Three case reports are given with recurrent psychoses of the bipolar form and with recurrent schizomanic psychoses. The course of the disease is pointed out, and the patients' treatment with a prophylactic medication is described. The three patients remain stable under this treatment, and, this is important to note, they are socially integrated.

Keywords: Bipolar form, carbamazepine, clozapine, deficiency condition, haloperidol, lithium, olanzapine, prognosis, prophylactic medication, quetiapine, recurrent psychosis, residual condition, schizodepressive psychosis, schizomanic psychosis, total remission.

2.1. INTRODUCTION

Schizoaffective disorder features both psychotic and affective symptoms. The schizophrenic symptoms may include paranoia, acoustic hallucinations, *e.g.,* comments, orders, an order to commit suicide, or voices talking to each other [1]. The affective symptoms may be monopolar, *e.g.,* they comprise manic symptoms such as hyperactivity, sleep disturbances, and megalomania, or depressive symptoms, such as prolonged sadness, decreased activity, sleep disturbances with early awakening, and depressive paranoia [1]. A bipolar form of the schizoaffective disorder is also possible, when depressive and manic symptoms occur alternatively.

It has been observed that the prognosis of schizoaffective disorder is better than that of schizophrenia [2]. It happens that in some cases the schizoaffective disorder is manifested by only one episode of acute psychosis, after which the psychotic and affective symptoms show complete remission [1]. If schizoaffective patients show a tendency towards recurrent disease symptoms, remission is still possible, and the course of the disease is more favorable than in schizophrenic patients [2]. The question as to why the schizoaffective disorder still has a favorable prognosis will be answered in the chapter discussing neural networks [1].

2.2. FORMS OF SCHIZOAFFECTIVE DISORDER

2.2.1. Schizoaffective Disorder with a Single Episode of Psychosis and Total Remission

Schizoaffective disorder has a better prognosis than schizophrenia [3]. Some patients develop a single episode of schizomanic or schizodepressive psychosis and then show total remission of their psychotic symptoms. Antipsychotic treatment is continued for some years, and no recurrence of the psychotic symptoms occurs [3]. The only symptom that remains in these patients is their vulnerability and sensitivity. Huber *et al.* [3] showed that this form of schizoaffective disorder includes one third of patients diagnosed with the disorder. These patients can usually be reintegrated into their professional and social lives. The question arises as to why single-episode schizoaffective disorder has a tendency to be accompanied by total remission of the psychotic symptoms. We shall try to find an answer to this puzzling issue by describing the neural networks in the affective and the mesolimbic systems that are able to reverse the neurotransmitter imbalance [2].

2.2.2. Schizoaffective Disorder with Recurrent Psychoses and a Residual Condition

The most frequent form of schizoaffective disorder is recurrent psychosis with a residual condition. Considering the three case reports of schizoaffective patients discussed below, all three individuals suffer from this form of the disease. The first patient shows schizophrenic symptoms with a bipolar form with recurrent psychoses (severe form); she was treated with clozapine and two mood-stabilizing drugs, *i.e.,* carbamazepine and lithium. The result was a severe residual condition, because after the first episode of psychosis, she was granted a state pension and no longer worked. She is socially reintegrated through her participation in a self-help group.

The second patient had recurrent episodes of schizomanic psychosis and, at the end, she had a residual condition. She also obtained a state pension and works part-time. The third patient also showed recurrent schizomanic psychoses and after some years, she obtained a semi-pension and has a part-time job. She also developed a residual condition and still has social problems, because she is unable to deal with her son, with whom she tends to get aggressive.

As indicated above, Huber and Gross [3] reported that one third of schizoaffective patients show recurrent episodes of psychosis with a residual condition. However, the patients show increasingly fewer severe basic symptoms than those occurring in schizophrenic patients [3]. Moreover, those authors found that the schizomanic form of schizoaffective disorder has a better prognosis than the form with bipolar affective, *i.e.,* depressive and manic symptoms [3]. In the chapter describing neural networks, it will be explained why the schizoaffective disorder has fewer residual symptoms than schizophrenia [2].

2.2.3. Schizoaffective Disorder with Recurrent Psychoses and a Deficiency Condition

Schizoaffective disorder with recurrent episodes of psychosis and a deficiency condition is rare because its prognosis is generally more favorable than that of schizophrenia [3]. In schizophrenia, about one third of patients show a deficiency condition. We report a 60-year old patient who still has recurrent episodes of psychosis and can only be treated with haloperidol, a D_2 antagonist. He showed no dyskinesia. He obtained a state pension and his efforts to keep a job were not successful because he developed aggressive behaviour. He was married to a woman with a psychotic illness but still remains in the relationship.

2.3. CASE REPORTS

2.3.1. Case Report 1: Recurrent Schizoaffective Disorder with a Bipolar Form

We report a 57 year-old-woman who was suffering from schizoaffective disorder with schizophrenic, depressive and manic symptoms. At the age of 27, she developed psychosis for the first time. She was married and had a 4-year-old daughter. She was working as kindergarten teacher and complained about insomnia and that she had difficulties in performing her work. She had persecution complex and heard voices talking to each other. At that time she was treated in a psychiatric ward. Her symptoms improved only slowly and the physicians decided to apply electroconvulsive therapy. She was treated with haloperidol, but this typical neuroleptic led to severe movement disturbances. After 18 months of treatment, she was treated with haloperidol (100 mg) in an injectable depot form and lithium as prophylactic medication [4]. As a consequence of the long treatment she retired. She divorced 6 years after the in-patient treatment and had difficulties in overseeing her daughter's education. She could fulfill her duties at home, but she suffered from depression, mania or paranoia from time to time. At the age of 43, she was admitted again to a psychiatric hospital. Since her complaints had not yet improved, the treatment was changed. She received 100 mg of clozapine, 600 mg of carbamazepine and 300 mg of lithium acetate [5, 6]. The atypical neuroleptic clozapine improved the psychotic symptoms notably. She still had depressive and manic symptoms from time to time. She joined a self-help group and has remained stable since that time.

2.3.2. Case Report 2: Recurrent Schizomanic Psychosis

We report a 66-year-old woman who for the first time showed psychotic and manic symptoms at the age of 28, after the death of her first child. She showed paranoid and manic symptoms and acoustic hallucinations. She spent two years in an in-patient ward and she retired after the treatment. She was reintegrated into social life and worked part-time again as a music teacher. She often underwent a recurrence of the psychotic and manic symptoms and had ideations of suicide. She was treated with clozapine (100 mg), after which the psychotic symptoms improved considerably. Ten years later, clozapine was replaced by quetiapine (400 mg), and as a result she became free of her acute psychotic and manic symptoms [7, 8]. She shows good adherence to her drug regimen and maintains social integration by participating actively in a self-help group.

2.3.3. Case Report 3: Recurrent Schizomanic Psychosis

We describe a 40-year-old woman who showed psychotic and manic symptoms for the first time at the age of 18. At that time, she was diagnosed with hebephrenia. She suffered at the hands of her very strict parents and studied dietetics in another town, but then underwent a recurrence of her psychotic and manic symptoms. She had a persecution complex and acoustic hallucinations, for which she was treated with haloperidol (8 mg). She started to work in her professional capacity, but then had to take partial retirement. Ten years later, she got married and gave birth to a son. She then developed two episodes of psychosis. She was first treated with ziprasidone (80 mg), but with this she began to develop suicidal ideations. From that time on, she received a treatment with olanzapine (10 mg) and remained stable [9]. Her mother-in-law took over her son's education, because she was socially intractable and aloof and was therefore unable to look after him. She is now working part-time as an adviser in dietetics.

REFERENCES

[1]   Klosterkötter, J. Indicated prevention of schizophrenia. Dtsch Arztebl Int 2008; 105: 532- 9.
[2]   Werner F-M, Coveñas R. Treatment of the schizoaffective disorder according to a neuronal network. Klin Neurophysiol 2012; 43:103-4.

[3]   Huber G, Gross G. The concept of basic symptoms in schizophrenic and schizoaffective psychoses. Recent Prog Med 1989; 80: 646-52.

[4]   Malhi GS, Tanious M, Coulston CM, Berk M. Potential mechanisms of action of lithium in bipolar disorder: current understanding. CNS Drugs 2013; 27: 135-53.

[5]   Constantine RJ, Andel R, McPherson M, Tandon R. The risks and benefits of switching patients with schizophrenia or schizoaffective disorder from two to one antipsychotic medication: a randomized controlled trial. Schizophr Res 2015; 166: 194-200.

[6]   Karoly R, Lenkey N, Juhasz AO, Vizi ES, Mike A. Fast- or slow-inactivated state preference of Na^+ channel inhibitors: a simulation and experimental study. PloS Compact Biol 2010; 6: e10000818.

[7]   Maher AR, Theodore G. Summary of the comparative effectiveness review on off-label use of atypical antipsychotics. J Manag Care Pharm 2012; 18: S1-20.

[8]   Amr M, Lakhan SE, Sanhan S, Al-Rhaddad D, Hassan M, Thiabh M, Shams T. Efficacy and tolerability of quetiapine *versus* haloperidol in first-episode schizophrenia: a randomized clinical trial. Int Arch Med 2013; 6: 47.

[9]   Huang CL, Hwang TJ, Chen YH, *et al.* Intramuscular olanzapine *versus* intramuscular haloperidol plus lorazepam for the treatment of acute schizophrenia with agitation: an open-label, randomized, controlled trial. J Formos Med Assoc 2015; 114: 438-45.

CHAPTER 3

Schizoaffective Disorder: Alterations of Neurotransmitters and Neuropeptides in Brain Centers Involved in Psychotic and Affective Symptoms

Abstract: Here, we describe the alterations of classical neurotransmitters and neuropeptides, acting at specific subreceptors, in the brain regions involved in affective and schizophrenic symptoms in the schizoaffective disorder. In schizophrenic symptoms, alterations of the postsynaptic excitatory neurotransmitters dopamine and serotonin and hypoactivity of the presynaptic inhibitory neurotransmitter GABA and of glutamate occur in the mesolimbic system, hippocampus and prefrontal cortex. Neuropeptides, such as neurotensin, cholecystokinin and substance P act as neuromodulators. In depressive symptoms, brain regions such as the brainstem, hypothalamus and hippocampus are involved. Serotonin, dopamine, acetylcholine, GABA and glutamate play an important role. Neuropeptides such as galanin, neuropeptide Y and substance P are involved in the pathophysiology of the affective symptoms. Because schizophrenic and affective symptoms can be enhanced by stressful events or traumatisms, the hypothalamic-adrenal axis and its efferent connections to the brainstem and hippocampus are considered. We suggest additional pharmacotherapies for the treatment of the disease interfering with specific subreceptors of the classical neurotransmitters and neuropeptides described.

Keywords: Acetylcholine, antipsychotic drug, brainstem, cholecystokinin, dopamine, galanin, gastrin-releasing peptide, gamma-aminobutyric acid, glutamate, hippocampus, hypothalamus, hypothalamic-adrenal axis, mood-stabilizing drug, neural network, neuropeptide Y, neurotensin, prefrontal cortex, serotonin, tachykinin, ventral tegmental area.

In schizoaffective disorder, both schizophrenic and affective symptoms occur at the same time. The mesolimbic system, the hippocampus and the prefrontal cortex are involved in these symptoms. After the dopamine and serotonin hypothesis had been proposed for these brain regions, where dopamine hyperactivity *via* D_2 receptors, and serotonin hyperactivity *via* 5-HT_{2A} receptors occur, a multi-neurotransmitter system was suggested [1]. Neurotransmitters such as GABA, which acts as a presynaptic inhibitor, and glutamate, which partly exerts a presynaptic inhibitory function, also play an important role in schizoaffective disorder. Moreover, the dysfunction of the hypothalamic-adrenal (HPA) axis, with altered cortisol levels and hyperactivity of the corticotropin-releasing hormone

Felix-Martin Werner and Rafael Coveñas

(CRH), has a disease-modulating effect because CRH hyperactivity is correlated with dopamine hyperactivity [2]. It is important to establish a relationship between the HPA axis and the neurotransmitter alterations because stressful events enhance patients' vulnerability and can worsen the schizophrenic symptoms [2].

3.1. SCHIZOAFFECTIVE DISORDER: ALTERATIONS OF NEUROTRANSMITTERS AND NEUROPEPTIDES IN THE HYPOTHALAMUS, MESOLIMBIC SYSTEM, HIPPOCAMPUS AND PREFRONTAL CORTEX

In schizophrenia, alterations of the postsynaptic neurotransmitters dopamine and serotonin, of the presynaptic neurotransmitter GABA, and of glutamate, which partly acts as a presynaptic inhibitor, can be found. These alterations are due to the function of the common susceptibility genes: neuregulin-1, dysbindin-1, GAD (glutamic acid decarboxylase) 67, COMT (catechol-O-methyl tranferase) and monoamine oxidase [1]. The neurons acting through these classical neurotransmitters form an altered multi-neurotransmitter system in the mesolimbic system, the hippocampus and the prefrontal cortex. Neuropeptides that exert a neuromodulatory effect can influence the dysfunction of these classical neurotransmitters. Since 33% of schizoaffective patients report childhood trauma, we stress the dysfunction of the HPA axis and the relationship between increased cortisol levels and increased concentrations of CRH, and between the hyperactivity of D_2 dopaminergic and 5-HT_{2A} serotonergic neurons [2, 3].

3.1.1. Traumatisation in One Third of the Schizoaffective Patients: Dysfunction of the Hypothalamic-Adrenal Axis in Psychotic Symptoms

Ruby *et al.* [3] found that 33% of patients with a psychotic disorder reported childhood trauma. Additionally, schizophrenic and schizoaffective patients showed a higher sensitivity and reactivity to stress [3]. In these patients, cortisol levels were augmented in 44.2% of the cases and significantly decreased in 5.2%; as a consequence, CRH levels were increased [3]. It has been reported that steroids cause neurotoxicity in the hypothalamus [2]. Abnormal cortisol levels are observed during the day, while morning cortisol levels are negatively correlated with emotional and sexual abuse [3]. Moreover, the dexamethasone test, which is not affected by the administration of steroids, is associated with negative and cognitive schizophrenic symptoms [3]. The recurrence of psychotic symptoms is associated with a 250% increase in cortisol levels, and decreased cortisol levels are combined with improved psychotic and negative symptoms [3].

A relationship between childhood trauma, *i.e.,* dysfunction of the HPA axis and increased cortisol levels, has been reported, and it is known that increased levels of CRH are related to different genes, *i.e.,* the serotonin transporter gene and the COMT gene, which encodes dopamine hyperactivity *via* decreased dopamine breakdown [2]. In the chapter describing the neural networks in the hypothalamus and hippocampus, it will be pointed out that CRH neurons elicit a high activity of GABAergic neurons, which due to the GAD 67 gene weakly inhibit D_2 dopaminergic neurons in the hippocampus [2]. Moreover, CRH neurons activate glutaminergic neurons, which owing to the neuregulin-1 and dysbindin-1 genes weakly inhibit 5-HT_{2A} serotonergic neurons *via* m5Glu receptors in the hippocampus [2]. Serotonergic hyperactivity, *via* 5-HT_{2A} receptors, is enhanced by the serotonin transporter gene [2].

3.1.2. Schizoaffective Disorder: Alterations of Classical Neurotransmitters in the Mesolimbic System, Hippocampus and Prefrontal Cortex

Since the dopamine and serotonin hypothesis was introduced [4], a multi-neurotransmitter system including dopamine and serotonin hyperactivity and GABA and glutamate hypoactivity has been proposed to exist in the mesolimbic system and hippocampus [5]. Susceptibility genes such as COMT and monoamine oxidase, which encode dopamine hyperactivity through decreased breakdown, GAD 67, which encodes a GABA deficiency in the hippocampus, and dysbindin-1 and neuregulin-1, which encode a glutamate hypoactivity *via* NMDA (n-methyl-D-aspartate) receptors, have been reported [6]. It has been described that these common genes encode psychotic symptoms that can be treated by administering second-generation antipsychotic drugs, whereas rare genes such as NRGN and ZNF804A might cause treatment-resistant schizophrenic symptoms [2]. It has also been reported that after the administration of MK-801, an NMDA antagonist, animals develop schizophrenia-like behaviour that can only be ameliorated by 5-HT_{2A} antagonists or risperidone, a combined D_2 and 5-HT_{2A} antagonist, but not by haloperidol, a D_2 antagonist [7]. In light of these results, the question arises as to how to treat schizomanic psychosis: it is important to determine whether the treatment of this form can be achieved by administering a second-generation antipsychotic drug and topiramate, a mood-stabilizing drug that exerts an NMDA antagonistic effect. There is no doubt that second-generation antipsychotic drugs, which are mostly combined D_2 and 5-HT_{2A} antagonists, should be administered to treat psychotic symptoms. Currently, the treatment of schizophrenic symptoms with the injectable form of aripiprazole, a partial D_2 agonist, a 5-HT_{1A} agonist and a 5-HT_{2A} antagonist, is recommended; this exerts a stronger effect in preventing the recurrence of psychotic symptoms [8].

Another issue to be explored is whether antipsychotic drugs that interfere with other subreceptors of classical neurotransmitters, for example $GABA_A$, NMDA, nicotinic cholinergic (alpha7 nAchR), metabotropic glutaminergic and $5\text{-}HT_7$ receptors, might or might not have an additional therapeutic effect [1].

3.1.2.1. Dopamine

In schizophrenia and in schizoaffective disorder dopamine hyperactivity *via* D_2 receptors occurs in the mesolimbic system, hippocampus and prefrontal cortex [1, 4]. Ermis *et al.* [9] determined the Val158Met gene polymorphisms in male schizophrenic patients with or without premorbid cannabis use. The authors found that schizophrenic patients with Val/Val genotype had a greater tendency to use cannabis and that their mean total positive and negative syndrome scale score (PANSS total score) was significantly higher than that seen in patients with the Met allele [9]. Consequently, psychotic patients with COMT gene polymorphisms develop more severe psychotic symptoms and have a greater tendency to use cannabis [9]. Dopamine hyperactivity can be enhanced by a reduced activity of the COMT or monoamine oxidase enzymes which, owing to the susceptibility genes, catalyze a reduced breakdown of dopamine and hence facilitate increased dopamine activity in the mesolimbic system and hippocampus [1]. In the chapter describing neural networks, it will be shown that in the mesolimbic system, owing to the GAD 67 gene, GABAergic neurons exert a weak presynaptic inhibition of D_2 dopaminergic neurons and enhance D_2 dopamine hyperactivity.

Second-generation antipsychotic drugs such as risperidone, olanzapine and quetiapine have a D_2 and $5\text{-}HT_{2A}$ antagonistic effect, while risperidone has a higher affinity for the D_2 receptor and olanzapine and quetiapine a higher affinity for the $5\text{-}HT_{2A}$ receptor [10].

One of the susceptibility genes for schizophrenic symptoms is neuregulin-1, since in the hippocampus the neuregulin-1/ErbB signaling network causes dopamine hyperactivity and activates D_4 receptors [11]. Clozapine, which has a D_3, D_4 and $5\text{-}HT_{2A}$ antagonistic effect, has a superior antipsychotic effect in spite of its side effects such as neutropenia and agranulocytosis [10]. The issue of the neural connection between neurons expressing D_2 and D_4 receptors will be addressed in the chapter focused on neural networks.

3.1.2.2. Serotonin

In schizophrenic patients, serotonin hyperactivity *via* $5\text{-}HT_{2A}$ receptors occurs in the mesolimbic system and hippocampus [5]. Alterations in serotonin level are mostly due to polymorphisms of the serotonin transporter gene [12]. There is certain evidence to suggest a direct interaction between 5-HT$_{2A}$ serotonergic and NMDA glutaminergic neurons in these brain areas, because in an animal model of schizophrenia NMDA antagonists such as MK-801 caused schizophrenia-like symptoms. These symptoms can be ameliorated with second-generation antipsychotic drugs such as risperidone or ritanserin, respectively 5-HT$_{2A}$ and 5-HT$_{2C}$ antagonists, but not with haloperidol, a D$_2$ antagonist [7]. Strzelecki *et al.* [13] studied a 23-year-old schizophrenic patient treated with quetiapine and citalopram. The authors also administered sarcosine, a co-NMDA agonist, *i.e.,* a glycine transporter type 1 inhibitor, at a dose of 2 g. The patient developed increased drive, libido and inner tension. He showed hypomanic symptoms. After a dosage reduction to 1 g sarcosine, the patient's negative and cognitive symptoms improved [13]. In the mesolimbic system and hippocampus, 5-HT$_{2A}$ serotonin hyperactivity could be due to a decreased presynaptic inhibition carried out by NMDA glutaminergic neurons [1].

Agonism at 5-HT$_{2C}$ receptors could ameliorate negative and cognitive schizophrenic symptoms. There are some data about (-)-MBP, a 5-HT$_{2C}$ agonist that simultaneously exerts antagonistic effects at the 5-HT$_{2A}$ and 5-HT$_{2B}$ receptors and shows promising therapeutic effects in models of psychosis induced by drugs such as clozapine [14]. Other authors have described the clinical effects of lurasidone, a novel second-generation antipsychotic drug that exerts a D$_2$, 5-HT$_{2A}$ and 5-HT$_7$ antagonistic effect and a 5-HT$_{1A}$ agonistic effect. Through the 5-HT$_{1A}$ agonistic and the 5-HT$_7$ antagonistic effect, it improves cognitive function in schizophrenic patients [15].

3.1.2.3. Gamma-aminobutyric Acid

Gamma-aminobutyric acid (GABA) is a presynaptic inhibitory neurotransmitter that acts *via* GABA$_A$ and GABA$_B$ receptors. In schizophrenia, GABA is dysfunctional in the mesolimbic system, hippocampus and prefrontal cortex [1]. Hypoactivity of GABAergic neurons, which is encoded in the susceptibility gene GAD 67, could contribute to D$_2$ dopamine hyperactivity in the mesolimbic system and hippocampus, because GABAergic neurons weakly inhibit D$_2$ dopaminergic neurons *via* GABA$_A$ receptors [5].

The concentrations of DA (dopamine), 3, 4-dihydroxyphenylacetic acid (DOPAC), GABA and glutamate have been examined in a drug-induced model of schizophrenia [16]. The experimental animals were divided into three groups. The first group received a subcutaneous injection of MK-801, an NMDA antagonist;

the second group received a chronic administration of MK-801, and the third group served as a control [16]. In the first two groups, the concentrations of DA, DOPAC, GABA and glutamate decreased. This finding is a clue about GABA dysfunction in schizophrenia [16]. Decreased GABA levels in the hippocampus and prefrontal cortex (PFC) are associated with attention deficits [17]. Electroencephalographic and magnetencephalographic abnormalities have been reported, *i.e.,* altered gamma-band (30-80 Hz) cortical activities, in patients with a schizoaffective bipolar disorder [18]. In schizoaffective patients, dysfunction of the GABA$_A$ receptor and its control over cortical pyramidal cells has been studied genetically [18]. In patients with a remitted schizoaffective bipolar disorder, an increased gamma-band was detected, reflecting an abnormal cortical inhibitory-excitatory balance [18].

mRNA and 65-kDa isoform protein glutamic acid decarboxylase levels have been explored in the PFC of schizophrenic and schizoaffective patients [19]. The authors found lower GAD 67 mRNA levels and decreased levels of the GAD protein in the PFC of schizoaffective patients and, in the same region in schizophrenic patients, lower GAD 67 mRNA levels and normal GAD protein levels [19]. One interpretation of this may be that in schizoaffective patients, who have better cognitive functions than schizophrenic patients, a down-regulation of the GAD 65 protein counteracts the down-regulation of the GAD 67 mRNA [19].

3.1.2.4. Glutamate

Glutamate mostly exerts an excitotoxic, postsynaptic excitatory effect and, partly, a presynaptic inhibitory effect on ionotropic receptors (NMDA, AMPA (D, L-alpha-amino-2, 3-dihydro-4-methyl-3-oxo-4-isoxazolepropanoic acid) and KA (kainate)) and on metabotropic glutaminergic receptors. In schizophrenia, glutamate is hypofunctional in the mesolimbic system, the hippocampus and the PFC owing to the dysbindin-1 and neuregulin-1 susceptibility genes [1, 6]. Gottschalk *et al.* [20] used an orthogonal system-based proteomic enrichment approach based on label-free liquid chromatography mass spectrometry to determine glutaminergic signalling and energy metabolism in the brain of schizophrenic, schizoaffective and affective patients. The authors found hypoactivity of presynaptic glutaminergic signalling in schizophrenia and hyperactivity of presynaptic glutaminergic signalling in major depression [20]. Considering that NMDA antagonists such as MK-801 can induce schizophrenia-like behaviour in an animal model of schizophrenia and that this can be ameliorated by 5-HT$_{2A}$ antagonists, the following neural network can be proposed: in schizophrenia, *i.e.,* in the mesolimbic system and the hippocampus, glutaminergic neurons weakly inhibit, *via* NMDA receptors, 5-HT$_{2A}$ serotonergic neurons, which therefore show high activity [1, 20].

Second-generation antipsychotic drugs, which are mostly D$_2$ and 5-HT$_{2A}$ antagonists, have few therapeutic effects on cognitive functions [21]. It has been suggested that a positive allosteric modulator of the NMDA receptor should be developed in order to improve cognitive functions in schizophrenic and schizoaffective patients [21]. In animal models of schizophrenia, altered levels of transcription factor specificity 4 (SP4) and 1 (SP1) proteins, which are regulated by the NMDA receptor, have been reported [22]. The authors examined SP4 and SP1 levels in post-mortem studies of the hippocampus of schizophrenic patients by immunoblot and quantitative RT-PCR. SP4 and SP1 levels were found to be increased in schizophrenic patients after the administration of MK-801 and after high doses of haloperidol and clozapine [22]. SP4 and SP1 levels were not altered after subacute administration of haloperidol or clozapine [22].

Metabotropic glutaminergic neurons are able to modulate the effect of ionotropic glutaminergic neurons [23]. The therapeutic effect of agonists of the metabotropic glutaminergic (mGlu) 2/3 or mGlu5 receptors as additional treatment of schizophrenia should be examined [23]. In this sense, glutaminergic neurons activate NMDA glutaminergic neurons *via* the mGlu2/3 receptor, and glutaminergic neurons could presynaptically inhibit 5-HT$_{2A}$ serotonergic neurons in the hippocampus *via* mGlu5 receptors [23].

3.1.2.5. Acetylcholine

Acetylcholine is a postsynaptic excitatory and presynaptic inhibitory neurotransmitter that acts at muscarinic cholinergic and nicotinic cholinergic receptors [1]. It has been reported that the extrapyramidal side effects of typical neuroleptics, above all, can be improved by GABA$_A$ agonists, NMDA antagonists and M$_4$ antagonists [24]. Moreover, it is known that M$_4$ antagonists exacerbate psychotic symptoms [24]. Accordingly, the issue arises as to whether agonism at M$_4$ receptors has an antipsychotic effect.

A novel positive allosteric modulator of the M$_4$ receptor has been developed: VU-0467154. This compound has been administered to rodents after the administration of MK-801, an NMDA antagonist [25]. VU-0467154 improved hyperlocomotion and the deficits in associative learning and memory and reversed the effects induced by MK-801 [25]. However, VU-0467154 failed to ameliorate the effects induced by MK-801 in M$_4$ knock-out mice [25]. In the PFC, an antagonistic interaction between D_1 dopaminergic neurons with a hyperactivity and M_4 muscarinic cholinergic neurons with a hypoactivity occurs [26]. Positive allosteric modulators of the M_4 receptor could enhance presynaptic GABAergic inhibition of D_1 dopaminergic neurons located in the PFC of schizophrenic patients and, to a lesser extent, in schizoaffective patients because GABAergic neurons show hypoactivity in the PFC of schizoaffective patients [19].

Cognitive deficits are common in schizophrenic patients and, although to a lesser extent, in schizoaffective patients, leading to increased disability [27]. A novel alpha7 nAChR partial agonist, EVP-6124, has been examined in schizophrenic and schizoaffective patients, who continued with second-generation antipsychotic drug treatment [27]. Cognitive test performances and event-related electroencephalographic (EEG) potentials revealed significantly better results in patients treated only with a second-generation antipsychotic drug [27]. This investigation should be continued with a view to developing nAChR agonists in order to improve cognitive function in schizophrenic and schizoaffective patients [27]. In the chapter focused on neural networks, it will be pointed out that nicotinic cholinergic neurons activate GABAergic neurons in the hippocampus *via* alpha7 nAch receptors and that, in the same central nervous region, nicotinic cholinergic neurons also activate D_2 dopaminergic neurons *via* alpha4beta2 nAch receptors [28].

3.1.3. Schizoaffective Disorder: Alterations of Neuropeptides in the Mesolimbic System, Hippocampus and Prefrontal Cortex

Neuropeptides act as neuromodulators, and altered levels of neuropeptides have been found in different brain regions in neurological and psychiatric diseases such as generalized epilepsy, Alzheimer's and Parkinson's disease, major depression and schizophrenia [29-33]. The question arises as to whether analogues, agonists or antagonists might be administered as additional therapy in schizoaffective disorder and whether these drugs might or might not improve the course of the disease [1, 32].

3.1.3.1. Cholecystokinin Involved in Chronic Auditory Hallucinations

In schizophrenic patients, cholecystokinin (CCK) levels have been found to be decreased in the striatum, nucleus accumbens, amygdala and frontal and temporal cortices, but are increased after treatment with neuroleptics in the striatum and the frontal and temporal cortices [34]. In a comparison with healthy volunteers, Basoglu *et al.* [35] examined the Brief Psychiatric Rating Scales, the Positive and

Negative Symptom Scores, the mass index, the lipid profile, and leptin, grhelin and cholecystokinin levels in schizophrenic patients with first-episode psychosis before and after 6 weeks of treatment with olanzapine. The authors found increases in the body mass index and in the lipid profile; however, neuropeptide levels showed no change after treatment with olanzapine. They found that in schizophrenic patients alterations in neuropeptide levels were due to alterations in dopamine and serotonin [35]. The interaction between CB_1 cannabinoid neurons and CCK neurons has been examined. In the PFC, an antagonistic interaction between CB_1 cannabinoid neurons and CCK neurons has been reported [35]. In the chapter focused on neural networks, it is explained that cannabinoid neurons strongly inhibit CCK neurons presynaptically *via* CB_1 receptors. CCK neurons transmit a weak activating impulse *via* CCK_A receptors to glutaminergic neurons, which weakly inhibit $5\text{-}HT_{2A}$ serotonergic neurons in the mesolimbic system *via* NMDA receptors [35].

In schizophrenic patients, an association between the gene for the CCK_A receptor and chronic auditory hallucinations has been reported [36]. Clinical trials should be carried out to explore whether CCK_A agonists or CB_1 antagonists might improve this disabling symptom in schizophrenic or schizoaffective patients [36, 37].

3.1.3.2. Corticotropin-releasing Factor

In the cerebrospinal fluid (CSF), corticotropin-releasing factor (CRF) levels are increased in schizophrenic patients [38]. Neuropeptide Y and CRF concentrations have been examined in the CSF of schizophrenic patients: neuropeptide Y levels increased and CRF levels decreased, and this was correlated with negative symptoms and anxiety [39]. It has been reported that 33% of schizophrenic and schizoaffective patients had undergone a childhood trauma [2]. Such trauma leads to a dysfunction of the HPA axis, and in most cases, cortisol and CRH levels are increased [2]. Moreover, these authors found a relationship between the HPA axis dysfunction and the increased dopamine and serotonin levels observed in the mesolimbic system and hippocampus. In the chapter focused on neural networks, it is pointed out that in the hypothalamus CRH neurons transmit an activating impulse *via* CRH_1 receptors to GABAergic and glutaminergic neurons. Owing to the expression of the GAD-67 gene, the GABAergic neurons weakly inhibit D_2 dopaminergic neurons located in the hippocampus presynaptically, and glutaminergic neurons weakly inhibit $5\text{-}HT_{2A}$ serotonergic neurons located in the hippocampus *via* mGlu5 receptors [2].

3.1.3.3. Dynorphin and Enkephalin

The kappa-opioid receptor dynorphin system is involved in the control of emotions, cognition and motivation and is dysfunctional in mood and psychotic disorders [40]. Some kappa-opioid receptor agonists might exert analgesic effects and improve cognitive function, although they produce side effects such as dysphoria, hallucinations and sedation [40]. However, some kappa-opioid receptor agonists that do not recruit the arrestin pathway have analgesic effects, without producing the above adverse effects [40]. It has been described that opioid receptor agonists have a slight antipsychotic effect, whereas opioid receptor antagonists may worsen the psychotic symptoms [41]. It has been reported that D_1 and D_2 receptors are localized in dynorphin/enkephalin neurons in the nucleus accumbens and in the basal ganglia, and above all in the globus pallidus [42]. In order to determine the existence of an antipsychotic effect of kappa-opioid receptor agonists, the effect of these drugs on prepulse inhibition of the acoustic startle reflex has been examined in an animal model of schizophrenia. It was reported that the prepulse inhibition induced by the NMDA antagonist MK-801 was not altered by kappa-opioid agonists or by kappa-opioid antagonists [43].

3.1.3.4. Galanin

In animal experiments in which schizophrenia-like symptoms were induced experimentally reduced galanin levels have been reported in the ventromedial and dorsomedial hypothalamus and in the lateral hypothalamic area [1]. Reduced galanin levels were also found in the CSF of schizophrenic patients [44].

The effect of intracerebrally administered galanin on dopaminergic neurotransmission in different brain areas has been explored [45]. The authors found that when administered into the ventral tegmental area galanin modulated the contents of l-dopa and 5-HT; however, administration into the nucleus accumbens had no modulating effect. Consequently, galanin neurons, located in the neostriatum, inhibit D_2 dopaminergic neurons in the mesolimbic system [45].

3.1.3.5. Gastrin-releasing Peptide

In an animal model of cognitive impairment, namely mice lacking the calcium/calmodulin-dependent protein kinase II alpha heterozygous knockout gene, it has been reported that the gastrin-releasing peptide gene is the most dysregulated one [46]. Owing to the lack of gastrin-releasing peptide, elevated neurogenesis and impaired neuronal development were observed; both phenomena were reversed when an intracerebroventricular infusion of the peptide was carried out. Consequently, gastrin-releasing peptide is essential for both adult hippocampal neurogenesis and normal neuronal development [46].

Gastrin-releasing peptide and its receptor (gastrin-releasing peptide receptor (GRPR)) are distributed throughout the CNS [47]. In schizophrenia, alterations in gastrin-releasing peptide have been found in the dorsal hippocampus and amygdala [47]. Therefore, gastrin-releasing peptide and its receptor could be novel targets in the treatment of schizophrenic symptoms [47]. In animal experiments, the GRP antagonist RC-3,095 may ameliorate the schizophrenic symptoms induced by a dopamine agonist, but not by an NMDA antagonist [48]. Consequently, in the mesolimbic system an interaction could occur between GRP neurons and D_2 dopaminergic neurons [48].

3.1.3.6. Neuropeptide Y

Neuropeptide Y is one of the hypothalamic hormones that increases appetite and leads to weight gain. Neuropeptide Y levels have been compared in schizophrenic patients treated with clozapine and in healthy subjects [49]. In both groups, the authors found no significant differences in the levels of neuropeptide Y [49].

In an animal model of schizophrenia, it has been examined whether the administration of the neuropeptide Y Y_2 agonist, named PYY (3-36), could cause schizophrenia-like behavior [50]. At low doses, PYY (3-36) impaired the social interaction of mice and at higher doses it led to a disruption of sensorimotor gating in the form of a prepulse inhibition deficiency [50]. The schizophrenia-like symptoms could be counteracted by haloperidol, a D_2 antagonist, but not by clozapine, a D_3, D_4 and $5\text{-}HT_{2A}$ antagonist. Consequently, in the mesolimbic system an interaction between Y_2 neuropeptide Y neurons and D_2 dopaminergic neurons could exist [50].

3.1.3.7. Neurotensin, the "Endogenous Neuropeptide"

Neurotensin is considered to be an endogenous neuroleptic because it exerts antipsychotic properties. Neurotensin levels are reduced in the mesolimbic system and the CSF of schizophrenic patients, but are augmented after neuroleptic treatment [51]. It is known that neurotensin neurons, located in the PFC, are connected to D_2 dopaminergic neurons of the mesolimbic system *via* presynaptic GABAergic neurons [52] and that neurotensin-like oligopeptides exert antipsychotic properties in animal models of schizophrenia. After schizophrenia-like symptoms had been induced by apomorphine injections, the neuropeptide-like oligopeptides influenced the dopaminergic system. Radioligand analysis revealed that these drugs compete with sulpiride, a D_2 and D_3 receptor antagonist, for blockade of the D_2 receptor [53]. Dilept, a neurotensin-like dipeptide, exerts a prestimulus inhibition (PSI) of the acoustic startle reflex in rats. Administered either as an injection or orally, Dilept exerted this effect in rats with schizophrenia-like symptoms induced by the NMDA antagonist ketamine [54].

Neurotensin exerts its effect on two subreceptors, the NTS_1 and NTS_2 receptors [55]. In experiments involving NTS_1 and NTS_2 knock-out wild-mice, it has been reported that activation of NTS_1 receptors antagonized the effect of psychotomimetic drugs, such as apomorphine, a D_2 agonist, and dizoclipine, an NMDA antagonist [55].

3.1.3.8. Oxytocin and Vasopressin

In schizophrenic patients, decreased oxytocin levels have been found in the amygdala, but its levels remain unchanged after antipsychotic treatment. In an animal model of schizophrenia, the administration of oxytocin was able to ameliorate social behaviour [56]. The relationship between the oxytocin pathway genes (OXT, OXTR, AVP, and CD38) and impaired social behaviour and susceptibility to psychotic disorders was explored in a large cohort of psychotic patients and healthy volunteers. While no association was found between the diagnosis of a psychotic disorder and the oxytocin pathway genes, these genes were correlated with dysfunction in social behaviour [57]. In schizophrenic patients, vasopressin levels have been found to be decreased in the temporal cortex. In an animal model of schizophrenia, the administration of vasopressin could improve deficits in social behaviour [58]. Since oxytocin has only weak effectiveness as an oral drug, the compound WAY-267,464, a vasopressin agonist acting at the vasopressin subreceptors V_{1a}, V_{1b} and V_2, was developed; in animal experiments, this agonist improved social behavior and exerted an anxiolytic effect [59, 60].

3.1.3.9. Peptide YY

Peptide YY has been examined in post-mortem investigations and was found in reduced concentrations in the temporal cortex, although in the hypothalamus its level was unchanged [60]. Moreover, in schizophrenic patients reduced peptide YY levels were found in the CSF [60].

3.1.3.10. Pituitary-adenylate Cyclase Activating Polypeptide

The pituitary-adenylate activating polypeptide (PACAP) is a risk gene for schizophrenia [61]. Mice with heterozygous disruption of the PACAP gene show behavioral abnormalities that can be ameliorated with risperidone, a D_2 and 5-HT_{2A} antagonist, or with ritanserin, a 5-HT_{2A} antagonist [61]. PACAP heterozygous mutant mice have been administered a 5-HT_{2A} agonist, the hallucinogenic drug ($\pm$)-2,5-dimethoxy-4-iodoamphetamine (DOI) [61]. After DOI administration, the animals showed greater head-twitch responses. DOI induced deficits in sensorimotor gating; other 5-HT_{2A} dependent responses were similar in PACAP(+/-) and wild-type mice [61]. The metabotropic glutaminergic (mGlu) 2/3 receptor is involved in the pathophysiology of schizophrenia [62]. MGS0028, an mGlu 2/3 receptor agonist, was administered to mice lacking PACAP [62]. MGS0028 improved the novel-object recognition test and other behavioral abnormalities in PACAP-deficient mice [62]. Accordingly, in schizophrenia PACAP must be involved in the hippocampal neural network and it would be connected to mGlu2/3 and 5-HT_{2A} serotonergic neurons [61, 62].

3.1.3.11. Secretin

Secretin is involved in the pathophysiology of schizophrenia, and reduced secretin CSF levels have been associated with symptoms of autism [1]. A clinical trial has been performed in which porcine secretin was administered intravenously along four weeks to patients suffering refractory schizophrenia; the results were compared with the control group (placebo) [63]. After secretin administration, the authors examined the PANSS (positive and negative syndrome scale) score. Although there were no significant differences between the group receiving secretin and the control group, some patients reported that the autistic symptoms had improved considerably [63].

3.1.3.12. Somatostatin

In the hippocampus, somatostatin is also involved in schizophrenia [64]. The number of interneurons and the number of somatostatin- and parvalbumin-positive interneurons in the hippocampus of schizophrenic patients in comparison to healthy subjects have been explored [64]. Although the number of interneurons was equal in both groups, the number of somatostatin- and parvalbumin-positive interneurons was reduced in the group of schizophrenic patients [64]. It has been shown that the transplantation of precursor cells of GABAergic interneurons into the medial PFC of mice prevents the induction of the cognitive and sensory-motor gating deficits induced by phencyclidine [65]. GABAergic interneurons can be sub-classified into somatostatin-/reelin-expressing interneurons. In an animal experiment, it has been shown that when injected into the lateral ventricle of mice reelin prevented cognitive and sensory-motor gating deficits after the administration of phencyclidine [65].

3.1.3.13. Tachykinins/substanceP

Tachykinins (substance P, neurokinin A and B) exert their effect *via* three subreceptors, namely the NK_1, NK_2 and NK_3 receptors. While substance P has elevated levels in major depression, neurokinin B activates D_2 dopaminergic neurons in the mesolimbic system *via* NK_3 receptors [32]. In schizophrenic patients, the efficacy of a selective, orally administered NK_3 receptor antagonist, named AZD2624 has been examined [66]. The patients were divided into three groups: the first was treated with AZD2624 for four weeks; the second group received a placebo, and the third group was administered olanzapine. After the four-week treatment, the PANSS score was measured, and cognition was evaluated with the CogState questionnaire. The authors found no differences between the second group receiving placebo and the group treated with AZD2624. Consequently, the NK_3 receptor antagonist AZD2624 does not improve either positive or negative schizophrenic symptoms, or cognitive functions [66].

3.1.3.14. Vasoactive Intestinal Peptide

Vasoactive intestinal peptide (VIP) and pituitary adenylate cyclase-activating polypeptide (PACAP) exert their effects on three subreceptors, PAC(1), VPAC(1) and VPAC(2) and have a neuroprotective effect in schizophrenia [67, 68]. While PACAP has a greater affinity for the PAC(1) receptor, VIP above all binds to the VPAC(1) and VPAC(2) receptors. The gene for the VPAC(2) receptor is a risk gene for schizophrenia, and the gene for the PAC(1) receptor is a risk gene for post-traumatic stress disorder [68].

3.2. SCHIZOAFFECTIVE DISORDER: ALTERATIONS OF CLASSICAL NEUROTRANSMITTERS AND NEUROPEPTIDES IN THE HYPOTHALAMUS, MIDBRAIN AND HIPPOCAMPUS

In schizoaffective patients, schizophrenic symptoms are accompanied by affective symptoms, *i.e.,* depressive, manic or bipolar, and alternating depressive and manic symptoms. In schizodepressive patients, monamine hypoactivity, *i.e.,* serotonin, noradrenaline and dopamine, has been found in the brainstem and hippocampus [1]. These neurotransmitter alterations are partly encoded by the monamine transporter genes [1]. Presynaptic inhibitory neurotransmitters such as glutamate and GABA are involved in the pathophysiology of depressive symptoms because, *via* $GABA_B$ receptors, GABAergic neurons strongly inhibit alpha1 noradrenergic neurons located in the brainstem and enhance noradrenaline deficiency [69]. *Via* mGlu5 receptors, glutaminergic neurons strongly inhibit $5\text{-}HT_{1A}$ serotonergic neurons and enhance serotonin hypoactivity in the brainstem [70, 71]. In the hippocampus, D_2 dopamine hypoactivity may also be associated with depressive symptoms [72]. In order to explain manic or bipolar behaviour, *i.e.,* alternating depressive and manic symptoms in schizoaffective patients, it is important to unravel the neural network in the hippocampus. This neural network includes the postsynaptic excitatory neurotransmitters dopamine and serotonin and the presynaptic inhibitory neurotransmitters GABA and glutamate [32].

3.2.1. Dysfunction of the Hypothalamic-Adrenocortical Axis in Affective Symptoms

A dysfunction of the hypothalamic-adrenocortical axis has been reported in depressive patients [73]. Enhanced responses in the dexamethasone (DEX)/corticotropin-releasing hormone (CRH) test have been recorded in depressive patients. Personality pathologies in correlation with the DEX/CRH test have been examined [73]. Suppressed cortisol responses were correlated with depressive symptoms, while other personality pathologies, such as schizoid, passive-aggressive or schizotypal, showed normal cortisol suppression after the DEX/CRH test [73]. It is known that the suppression of cortisol levels and the increase in CRH are correlated with the plasma concentrations of antidepressant drugs [74]. Might there be some relationship between the HPA axis and the neurotransmitters involved in depressive symptoms in the brainstem? CRH_1 receptor antagonists could have antidepressive effects. In the hypothalamus, CRH neurons transmit a strong activating impulse *via* CRH_1 receptors to glutaminergic neurons, which strongly inhibit $5\text{-}HT_{1A}$ serotonergic neurons located in the brainstem *via* m5Glu receptors [32]. The clinical effect of CRH_1 receptor antagonists will be addressed in another chapter.

3.2.2. Schizoaffective Disorder: Alterations of Classical Neurotransmitters in the Midbrain and Hippocampus

In schizoaffective disorder, the depressive and manic symptoms are localized in the brainstem and hippocampus. The main neurotransmitter alterations in the depressive symptoms have been described above. In manic symptoms, above all dopamine hyperactivity *via* D_2 receptors occurs in the hippocampus [32]. GABAergic neurons weakly inhibit D_2 dopaminergic neurons *via* $GABA_A$ receptors. GABA hypoactivity has been reported in schizoaffective disorder [19].

3.2.2.1. Serotonin

Among depressive symptoms, monamine hypoactivity, *i.e.,* serotonin, noradrenaline and dopamine, is found in the brainstem and hippocampus. In the dorsal raphe nucleus, the hypoactivity of serotonin is mediated by 5-HT$_{1A}$ receptors and may partly be due to polymorphisms of the 5-HT transporter gene. Both 5-HT$_{1A}$ agonists and SSRIs (selective serotonin reuptake inhibitors) may improve depressive symptoms [32]. Using the Hamilton Rating Scale for Depression, the antidepressive effects of SSRIs, such as citalopram, paroxetine and fluoxetine, were tested in comparison to placebo and this clinical trial showed that SSRIs did not have a significantly better effect than placebo, although a consistent superiority of SSRIs was found when depressed mood was the criterion examined [75]. An activation or blockade of other serotonin subreceptors, *i.e.,* a 5-HT$_{2C}$ agonistic effect or a 5-HT$_7$ antagonistic effect in the hippocampus, could contribute to the antidepressive effect of SSRIs [32]. Viladozone, a new antidepressive drug that exerts partial 5-HT$_{1A}$ agonism and inhibits serotonin reuptake, exerts a good antidepressive effect for the treatment of comorbid anxiety and has fewer sexual side effects [76]. It might be possible to enhance the antidepressive effect of SSRIs by administering NMDA antagonists or m5Glu antagonists [77]. In the brainstem, glutaminergic neurons strongly inhibit 5-HT$_{1A}$ serotonergic neurons *via* m5Glu receptors. In the hippocampus, *via* NMDA receptors glutaminergic neurons strongly inhibit 5-HT$_{2C}$ serotonergic neurons [32]. Consequently, antagonism at specific glutamate receptors might further enhance serotonergic neurotransmission [32, 77].

3.2.2.2. Noradrenaline

Noradrenaline (NA) is involved in the pathophysiology of depressive and manic symptoms in schizoaffective patients. In depressive patients, NA hypoactivity has been reported in the brainstem, with a reduced activation of alpha1 noradrenergic receptors [32]. NA hypoactivity is partly due to polymorphisms of the NA transporter gene, and patients with these polymorphisms respond better to selective serotonin and noradrenaline reuptake inhibitors than to SSRIs [72]. Depressive patients treated with duloxetine, a selective noradrenaline reuptake inhibitor, have been explored, using structural and functional MRI methods [78]. With this methodology, the authors observed increased hippocampal volume, which predicted a therapeutic response to duloxetine [78]. Adjunct treatment with edivoxetine, a highly selective noradrenaline reuptake inhibitor, was tested in 238 patients with a major depressive disorder, but these patients only responded partially to treatment with an SSRI [79]. Moderate improvements were observed on the Montgomery-Asberg Depression Rating Scale as from week 54. Adverse effects occurred in 5% of patients, while the main increases were found in systolic and diastolic blood pressure and heart rate [79].

3.2.2.3. Dopamine

Dopamine shows hypoactivity *via* D_2 receptors in the hippocampus of schizodepressive patients and hyperactivity in the hippocampus of schizomanic patients [1]. In a $[^{123}I]\beta$-CIT Spect study, serotonin and dopamine transporter availabilities in 27 depressive patients were examined before and after the administration of escitalopram [80]. Under treatment with escitalopram, an SSRI, occupancy in the thalamus for the serotonin transporter was 42%, whereas occupancy of the dopamine transporter was 25% [80]. Bupropion, a selective noradrenaline and dopamine reuptake inhibitor, increases symptoms such as decreased energy, interest and pleasure, and exerts a good antidepressant effect in depressive patients [81]. However, it is advisable not to administer bupropion in schizoaffective patients, because in schizomanic symptoms dopamine hyperactivity can occur in the mesolimbic system or the hippocampus and hence bupropion may enhance the schizomanic symptoms [1].

3.2.2.4. Acetylcholine

Acetylcholine is also involved in the pathogenesis of affective symptoms in schizoaffective disorder. Acetylcholine exerts its effect on muscarinic and nicotinic cholinergic receptors [1]. The activation of nicotinic cholinergic subreceptors could have antidepressive properties. Agonism at alpha4beta2 nAch receptors could exert an antidepressive effect, since these nicotinic cholinergic receptors activate dopaminergic neurons located in the hippocampus [82]. According to Rahman *et al.* [83], future studies should look at whether agonists at nicotinic cholinergic receptors, for example mecamylamine, an alpha7 nAch receptor agonist, or lobeline, an alpha4beta2 nAch receptor agonist, improve major depressive disorder in patients with comorbid alcohol or nicotine addiction [83].

3.2.2.5. Gamma-aminobutyric Acid

In affective symptoms, gamma-aminobutyric acid (GABA) is dysfunctional [84]. The presynaptic effect of GABA is mediated *via* $GABA_A$ and $GABA_B$ receptors. In the brainstem, the four neurotransmitters 5-HT, noradrenaline, GABA and glutamate form neural networks that play important roles in the circadian rhythm and as a "mood center" [77]. In the dorsal raphe nucleus, GABAergic neurons can strongly inhibit alpha1 noradrenergic neurons *via* $GABA_B$ receptors, enhancing noradrenaline deficiency, involved in depressive symptoms [69]. As a result, $GABA_B$ receptor antagonists should be examined in clinical trials in order to confirm their antidepressive effects [85]. Moreover, selective noradrenalin reuptake inhibitors should be combined with $GABA_B$ antagonists in order to obtain a stronger antidepressant effect [77]. In manic symptoms, GABAergic neurons might weakly inhibit D_2 dopaminergic neurons located in the hippocampus *via* $GABA_A$ receptors [32].

3.2.2.6. Glutamate

Glutamate is the main excitotoxic, *i.e.,* postsynaptic excitatory and partly presynaptic, inhibitory neurotransmitter and exerts its effect on ionotropic, *i.e.,* N-methyl-D-aspartate receptors and on metabotropic glutaminergic receptors [1]. In schizoaffective disorders, glutamate elicits hypo- and hyperactivity in the brain centers involved in affective symptoms [1]. It has been shown that glutaminergic neurons strongly inhibit $5-HT_{1A}$ serotonergic neurons in the brainstem *via* NMDA receptors. In the "mood center" of the brainstem, glutaminergic neurons strongly inhibit $5-HT_{1A}$ serotonergic neurons *via* m5Glu receptors [1]. Because these neurotransmitter alterations are correlated with depressive symptoms, the question arises as to whether NMDA antagonists or m5GluR antagonists can improve depressive symptoms. To a large extent, ketamine, an NMDA receptor antagonist, can improve depressive symptoms in sub-anesthetic-dose infusion but psychotomimetic effects should not be overlooked [86]. NMDA receptor antagonists should not be administered in schizodepressive patients because antagonism at NMDA receptors can enhance psychotic symptoms in the mesolimbic system [1]. However, clinical trials examining the antidepressive effect of m5GluR antagonists, for example MTEP, should be carried out [87].

3.2.3. Schizoaffective Disorder: Alterations of Neuropeptides in Midbrain and Hippocampus

In schizoaffective patients, some neuropeptides show alterations in the brain areas involved in affective symptoms. For example, in these patients galanin, neuropeptide Y and thyrotropin-releasing peptide elicit hypoactivity, whereas substance P elicits hyperactivity [1]. Clinical trials should be carried out to determine whether galanin agonists, neuropeptide Y agonists, thyrotropin-releasing hormone analogues or substance P antagonists exert antidepressive properties or not [1].

3.2.3.1. Galanin

In an animal model of major depression, mRNA levels of galanin were found to be decreased in the medial and lateral hypothalamus [88]. These levels increased after treatment with an SSRI [88]. Plasma galanin levels have been examined in patients with major depression, in patients in remission, and in healthy volunteers

[89]. Those authors also measured the Hamilton Rating Scale for Depression (HRSD) in depressive patients and in healthy volunteers. They found increased plasma galanin levels in depressive patients in comparison with healthy volunteers, together with a significant correlation between increased plasma galanin levels and the severity of the depressive symptoms and the score on the HRSD [89]. The question of whether galanin agonists, for example galanin 2 receptor agonists, could ameliorate depressive symptoms should be examined in clinical trials, because galanin neurons, originating in the hypothalamus, activate serotonergic neurons located in the hippocampus *via* Gal2 receptors [77, 88].

3.2.3.2. Neuropeptide Y

In depressive patients, neuropeptide Y (NPY) levels are decreased or increased after antidepressive treatment [74]. The question arises as to whether the administration of NPY analogues or NPY agonists exerts antidepressive properties. In a rodent model of single prolonged stress, it has been examined whether intranasal administration of NPY and/or of the melanocortin receptor four (MC4R) antagonist HS014 might have anxiolytic and antidepressant effects [90]. The authors found that in this animal model the intranasal administration of NPY, and to a greater extent HS014, had anxiolytic and antidepressant effects [90]. In the chapter addressing neural networks, it is pointed out that NPY neurons, originating in the dentate gyrus, activate GABAergic neurons located in the hippocampus *via* NPY$_1$ receptors [77].

3.2.3.3. Substance P

Substance P levels in the CSF are found to be increased in depressive patients and to be decreased after successful antidepressive pharmacotherapy [91]. In an animal model of depression, the antidepressant effect of substance P antagonists has been examined [92]. The authors injected substance P antagonists into the lateral habenula of rats with depressive-like behavior and found a therapeutic effect, with improved parameters in the forced swim-test [92]. Furthermore, increased 5-HT levels were found in the dorsal raphe nucleus after the administration of substance P antagonists [92]. In the chapter on the neural networks, it is remarked that substance P neurons activate GABAergic neurons located in the hippocampus *via* NK$_1$ receptors [77].

3.2.3.4. Thyrotropin-releasing Hormone

The administration of thyrotropin-releasing hormone (TRH) exerts a transient antidepressive effect [32]. Both the TRH and the DEX/CRH tests have been explored in patients in full remission from major depression [93]. In contrast to the DEX/CRH test, the TRH test did have a predictive value for the recurrence of major depression [93].

REFERENCES

[1]   Werner FM, Coveñas R. Classical neurotransmitters and neuropeptides involved in schizophrenia: How to choose the appropriate antipsychotic drug? Curr Drug Ther 2013; 8: 132-43.

[2]   Haller SC, Padmanabhan JL, Lizano P, Torous J, Keshavan M. Recent advances in understanding schizophrenia. F1000 Prime Reports 2014; 6: 57.

[3]   Ruby E, Polito S, McMahon K, Gorovitz M, Corcoran C, Malaspina D. Pathways associating childhood trauma to the neurobiology of schizophrenia. Front Psychol Behav Sci 2014; 3: 1-17.

[4]   Davidson M, Keffe RS, Mohs RC, et al. L- dopa challenge and relapse in schizophrenia. Am J Psychiatry 1987; 144: 934-8.

[5]   Werner FM. Schizophrenia: from the genetic localization to the cellular mechanism. Klin Neurol 2006; 37: 19-20.

[6]   Collier DA, Li T. The genetics of schizophrenia: glutamate not dopamine? Eur J Pharmacol 2003; 480: 177-84.

[7]   Nilsson M, Waters S, Waters N, Carlsson A, Carlsson ML. A behavioural pattern analysis of hypoglutaminergic mice-effects of four different antipsychotic agents. J Neural Transm 2001; 108: 1181-96.

[8]   Raoufinia A, Baker RA, Eramo A, et al. Initiation of aripiprazole once-monthly in patients with schizophrenia. Curr Res Med Opin 2015; 31: 583-92

[9]   Ermis A, Erkiran M, Dasdemir S, et al. The relationship between catchol-o-methyltransferase gene Val158Met (COMT) polymorphism and premorbid cannabis use in Turkish male patients with schizophrenia. In vivo 2015; 29: 129-32.

[10] Werner FM, Coveñas R. Safety of antipsychotic drugs: focus on therapeutic and adverse effects. Exp Opin Drug Saf 2014; 13: 1031-42.

[11] Andersson RH, Johnston A, Herman PA, et al. Neuregulin and dopamine modulation of hippocampal gamma oscillations is dependent on dopamine D4 receptors. Proc Natl Acad Sci USA 2012; 109: 13118-23.

[12] Aas M, Djurovic S, Athanasiu L, et al. Serotonin transporter gene polymorphism, childhood trauma, and cognition in patients with psychotic disorders. Schizophr Bull 2011; 38: 15-22.

[13] Strzelecki D, Szyburska J, Rabe-Jablonska J. Two grams of sacosine in schizophrenia – is it too much? A potential role of glutamte-serotonin interaction. Neuropsychiatr Dis Treat 2014; 10: 263-6.

[14] Canal CE, Morgan D, Felsing D, et al. A novel aminotetralin-type serotonin (HT) 2C receptor-specific agonist and 5-HT2A competitive antagonist/5-HT2B inverse agonist with clinical efficacy for psychoses. J Pharmacol Exp Ther 2014; 349: 310-8.

[15] Samalin L, Garnier M, Llorca PM. Clinical potential of lurasidone in the management of schizophrenia. Ther Clin Risk Manag 2011; 7: 239-50.

[16] Liu Y, Tang Y, Pu W, Zhang X, Zhao J. Concentration of DA, Glu and GABA in brain tissues in schizophrenia developmental model rats induced by MK-801. Zhong Nan Da Xue Xue Bao Yi Ban 2011; 36: 712-9.

[17] Paine TA, Slipp LE, Carlezon WA Jr. Schizophrenia-like attentional deficits following blockade of prefrontal cortex GABAA receptors. Neuropsychopharmacology 2011; 36: 1703-13.

[18] Brealy JA, Shaw A, Richardson H, Singh KD, Muthukumaraswamy SD, Keedwall PA. Increased visual gamma power in schizoaffective bipolar disorder. Psychol Med 2015; 45: 783-94.

[19] Glausier JR, Kimoto S, Fish KN, Lewis DA. Lower glutamic acid decarboxylase 65-kDa isoform messenger RNA and protein levels in the prefrontal cortex in schizoaffective disorder but not in schizophrenia. Bio Psychiatry 2015; 77: 167-76.

[20] Gottschalk MG, Wesseling H, Guest PC, Bahn S. Proteomic enrichment analysis of psychotic and affective disorders reveals common signatures in presynaptic glutamatergic signaling and energy metabolism. Int J Neuropsychopharmacol 2014; 18: 1-11.

[21]   Modhaddam B, Javitt D. From revolution to evolution: the glutamate hypothesis of schizophrenia and its implication for treatment. Neuropsychopharmacology 2011; 37: 4- 15.

[22]   Pinacho R, Valdiazán M, Pilar-Cuellar F, *et al*. Increased SP4 and SP1 transscription factor expression in the postmortem hippocampus of chronic schizophrenia. J Psychiatr Res 2014; 58: 189-96.

[23]   Vinson PN, Conn PJ. Metabotropic glutamate receptors as therapeutic targets for schizophrenia. Neuropharmacology 2011; 62: 1461-72.

[24]   Werner FM. Therapiemöglichkeiten medikamentös bedingter extrapyramidal bedingter Störungen. Neurol. Int. Akt-I 2008; 206. (www.anim2008.de).

[25]   Bubser M, Bridges TM, Dencker D, *et al*. Selective activation of M4 muscarinic acetylcholine receptors reveres MK- 801-induced behavioral impairments and enhances associative learning in rodents. ACS Chem Neurosci 2014; 5: 920-42.

[26]   Dencker D, Wörtwein G, Weikop P, *et al*. Involvement of a subpopulation of neuronal M4 muscarinic acetylcholine receptors in the antipsychotic-like effects of the M1/M4 preferring muscarinic receptor agonist xanomeline. J Neurosci 2011; 31: 5905-8.

[27]   Preskorn SH, Gawryl M, Dgetluck N, *et al*. Normalizing effect of EVP-6124, an alpha-7 nicotinic partial agonist, on event-related potentials and cognition: a proof of concept, randomized trial in patients with schizophrenia. J Psychiatr Pract 2014; 20: 12-24.

[28]   Wallace TL, Porter RH. Targeting the nicotinic alpha7 acetylcholine receptor to enhance cognition in disease. Biochem Pharmacol 2011; 81: 891-903.

[29]   Werner FM, Coveñas R. Neuropeptides and classical neurotransmitters involved in Parkinson and Alzheimer diseases. In: Coveñas R, Mangas A, Nárvaez JA, Eds. Focus on neuropeptide research; Trivandrum, Transworld Research Network 2007; pp. 299- 399.

[30]   Werner FM, Coveñas R. Classical neurotransmitters and neuropeptides involved in major depression: a review. Int J Neurosci 2010; 120: 455-70.

[31]   Werner FM, Coveñas R. Classical neurotransmitters and neuropeptides involved in generalized epilepsy: a focus on antiepileptic drugs. Curr Med Chem 2011; 18: 4933- 48.

[32]   Werner FM, Coveñas R. Classical neurotransmitters and neuropeptides involved in major depression in a multi-neurotransmitter system: focus on antidepressant drugs. Curr Med Chem 2013; 20: 4853-8.

[33]   Werner FM, Coveñas R. Review: Classical neurotransmitters and neuropeptides involved in generalized epilepsy in a multi-neurotransmitter system: How to improve the antiepileptic effect? Epilepsy Behav 2015; doi: 10.1016/j.yebeh.2015.01.038.

[34]   O'Connor WT. Functional neuroanatomy of the ventral striopallidal GABA pathway. new sites of intervention in the treatment of schizophrenia. J Neurosci Methods 2001; 109: 31-9.

[35]   Basoglu C, Oner O, Ates AM, Algul A, Semiz UB, Ebrinc S, Cetin M, Ozcan O, Iipcioglu OM. Association between symptom improvement and change of body mass index, lipid profile, and leptin, grhelin and cholecytokinin levels during 6-week olanzapine treatment in patients with first-episode psychosis. J Clin Psychopharmacol 2010; 30:636-8.

[36]   Eggan SM, Melchitzky DS, Sesack SR, Fish KN, Lewis DA. Relationship of cannabinoid CB1 receptor and cholecystokinin immunoreactivity in monkey dorsolateral prefrontal cortex. Neuroscience 2010; 169: 1652-61.

[37]   Sanjuan J, Toirac I, González JC, *et al*. A possible association between the CCK-AR gene and persistent auditory hallucinatons in schizophrenia. Eur Psychiatry 2004; 19: 349-53.

[38]   Werner FM, Coveñas R. Neuropeptides involved in schizophrenia. Curr Top Neurochem 2005; 4: 35-49.

[39]   Nikisch G, Baumann P, Liu T, Mathé, AA. Quetiapine affects neuropeptide Y and corticotropin-releasing hormone in cerebrospinal fluid from schizophrenia patients: relationship to depression and anxiety symptoms and to treatment response. Int J Neuropsychopharmacol 2011; 15: 1051-61.

[40]   White KL, Scopton AP, Rives ML, *et al*. Identification of novel functionally κ-opioid receptor scaffolds. Mol Pharmacol 2014; 85: 83-90.

[41]   Weatherspoon JK, González-Alvear GM, Frank AR, Werling LL. Regulation of [3H] dopamine release from mesolimbic and mesocortical areas of guinea pig brain by sigma receptors. Schizophr Res 1996; 21: 51-62.

[42] Perreault ML, Hasbi A, Alijaniaram M, *et al.* The dopamine D1-D2 receptor heteromer localizes in dynorphin/enkephalin neurons: increased high affinity state following amphetamine and in schizophrenia. J Biol Chem 2010; 19: 36625-34.

[43] Tejeda HA, Chefer VI, Zapata A, Shippenberg TS. The effects of kappa-opioid receptor ligands on prepulse inhibition and CRF-induced prepulse inhibition deficits in the rat. Psychopharmacology (Berl) 2010; 210: 231-40.

[44] Frederiksen SO, Ekman R, Gottfries CG, Widerlov E, Jonsson S. Reduced concentrations of galanin, arginine vasopressin, neuropeptide Y and peptide YY in the temporal cortex but not in the hypothalamus of brains from schizophrenics. Acta Psychiatr Scand 1991; 83: 273-7.

[45] Ericson E, Ahlenius S. Suggestive evidence for inhibitory effects of galanin on mesolimibic dopaminergic neurotransmission. Brain Res 1999; 822: 200-9.

[46] Walton NM, de Koning A, Xie X, *et al.* Gastrin-releasing contributes to the regulation of adult hippocampal neurogenesis and neuronal development. Stem Cells 2014; 32: 2545-66.

[47] Roesler R, Henriques JA, Schwartsmann G. Gastrin-releasing peptide receptor as a molecular target for psychiatric and neurological disorders. CNS Neurol Disord Drug Targets 2006; 5: 197-204.

[48] Meller CA, Henriques JA, Schwartsmann G, Roesler R. The bombesin/gastrin releasing peptide receptor antagonist RC-3095 blocks apomorphine but not MK-801-induced stereotypy in mice. Peptides 2004; 25: 585-8.

[49] Wysokinski A. Fasting serum levels of neuropeptide Y in patients with schizophrenia on clozapine monotherapy. Clin Neuropharmacol 2015; 38: 18-22.

[50] Stadlbauer U, Langhans W, Meyer U. Administration of the Y2 receptor agonist PYY 3-36 in mice induces multiple behavioral changes relevant to schizophrenia. Neuropsychopharmacology 2013; 38: 2446-55.

[51] Caceda R, Kinkead B, Nemeroff CB. Do neurotensin receptor agonists represent a novel class of antipsychotic drugs? Semin Clin Neuropsychiatry 2003; 8: 94-108.

[52] Kitagbi P. Targeting neurotensin receptors with agonists and antagonists for therapeutic purposes. Curr Opin Drug Discov Devel 2002; 5: 764-76.

[53] Kost NV, Meshavkin NV, Batshcheva Elu, Sokolov Olu, Andreeva AL, Miasoedev NF. Neurotensin-like oligopeptides as potential antipsychotics: effect on dopamine system. Eksp Klin Farmakol 2011; 74: 3-6.

[54] Ostrovskaia RU, Krupina NA, Gudasheva TA, Voronina TA, Seredenin SB. Neurotensin dipeptide analog dilept decreases the deficiency prestimulus startle reflex inhibition: a prognostic sign of antipsychotic activity. Eksp Klin Farmakol 2009; 72: 3-7.

[55] Oliveros A, Heckman MG, Del Pilar Corena-McLeod M, Williams K, Boules M, Richelson E. Sensorimotor gating in NTS1 and NTS2 null mice: effects of d- amphetamine, dizocilpine and NT69L. J Exp Biol 2010; 213: 4232-9.

[56] Feifel D, Reza T. Oxytocin modulates psychotomimetic-induced deficits in sensorimotor gating. Psychopharmacology (Berl) 1999; 141: 93-8.

[57] Haram M, Tesli M, Bettella F, Djurovic S, Andreassen OA, Melle I. Association genetic variation in the oxytocin receptor gene and emotional withdrawal, but not between oxytocin pathway genes and diagnosis in psychotic disorders. Front Hum Neurosci 2015; 9: 9.

[58] Elman I, Lukas S, Shoaf SE, Rott D, Adler C, Breier A. Effects of acute metabolic stress on the peripheral vasopressinergic system in schizophrenia. J Psychopharmacol 2003; 17: 317-23.

[59] Ring RH, Schechter LE, Leonard SK, *et al.* Receptor and behavioral pharmacology of WAY-267,464, a non-peptide oxytocin receptor agonist. Neuropharmacology 2010; 58: 69-77.

[60] Frederiksen SO, Ekman R, Gottfries CG, Widerlov E, Jonsson S. Reduced concentrations of galanin, arginine vasopressin, neuropeptide Y and peptide YY in the temporal cortex but not in the hypothalamus of brains from schizophrenics. Acta Psychiatr Scand 1991; 83: 273-7.

[61] Hazama K, Hayata-Takano K, Uetsuki K, *et al.* Increased behavioral and neuronal responses to a hallucinogenic drug in PACAP heterozygous mutant mice. PLos One 2014; 9: e89153.

[62] Ago Y, Hiramatsu N, Ishihama T, *et al.* The selective metabotropic glutamtae 2/3 receptor agonist MGS0028 reverses psychomotor abnormalities and recognition memory deficits in mice lacking the pituitary adenylate cyclase-activating polypeptide. Behav Pharmacol 2013; 24: 74-7.

[63] Sheitman BB, Knable MB, Jarskog LF, *et al.* Secretin for refractory schizophrenia. Schizophr Res 2004; 66: 177-81.

[64]   Konradi C, Yang CK, Zimmermann EL, *et al.* Hippocampal interneurons are abnormal in schizophrenia. Schizophre Res 2011; 131: 165-73.

[65]   Ishii K, Nagai T, Hirota Y, *et al.* Reelin has a preventive effect on phencyclidine-induced cognitive and sensory-motor gating deficits. Neurosci Res 2015; 96: 30-6.

[66]   Litman RE, Smith MA, Desai DG, Simpson T, Sweitzer D, Kanes SJ. The selective neurokinin 3 antagonist AZD2624 does not improve symptoms or cognition in schizophrenia: a proof-of-principle study. J Clin Psychopharmacol 2014; 34: 199- 204.

[67]   Moody TW, Ito T, Osefo N, Jensen RT. VIP and PACAP: recent insight into their functions/roles in physiology and disease from molecular and genetic studies. Curr Opin Endocrinol Diabetes Obes 2011; 18: 61-7.

[68]   Harmar AJ, Fahrekrug J, Gozes I, *et al.* Pharmacology and functions of receptors for vasoactive intestinal peptide and pituitary adenylate cyclase-activating polypeptide: IUPHAR review 1. Br J Pharmacol 2012; 166: 4-17.

[69]   Nowak G, Partyka A, Palucha A, *et al.* Antidepressant-like activity of CGP 36742 and CGP 51176, selective GABAB receptor antagonists, in rodents. Br J Pharmacol 2006; 159: 581-90.

[70]   Sanacora G, Kendell SF, Levin Y, *et al.* Preliminary evidence of riluzole efficacy in antidepressant-treated patients with residual depressive symptoms. Biol Psychiatry 2007; 61: 822-5.

[71]   Palucha A. Are compounds acting at metabotropic glutamate receptors the answer to treating depression? Expert Opin Invest Drugs 2006; 15: 1545-53.

[72]   Nutt DJ, Demytttenaere K, Janka K, *et al.* The other face of depression, reduced positive effect: the role of catecholamines in causation and cure. J Psychopharmacol 2007; 21: 461-71.

[73]   Schweitzer I, Tuckwell V, Maguire K, Tiller J. Personality pathology, depression and HPA functioning. Hum Psychopharmacol 2001; 16: 303-8.

[74]   Nikisch G, Agren H, Eap CB, Czernik A, Baumann P, Mathe AA. Neuropeptide Y and corticotropin-releasing hormone in CSF mark response to antidepressant treatment with citalopram. Neuropsychopharmacology 2005; 8: 403-16.

[75]   Hieronymus F, Emisson JF, Nilsson S, Eriksson E. Consistent superiority of selective serotonin reuptake inhibitors over placebo in reducing depressed mood in patients with major depression. Mol Psychiatry 2015; doi: 10.1038/mp.2015.53.

[76]   Hellerstein DJ, Flaxer J. Vilazodone for the treatment of major depressive disorder: an evidence-based review on its place in the therapy. Core Evid 2015; 10: 49-62.

[77]   Werner FM, Coveñas R. Classical neurotransmitters and neuropeptides involved in major depression: a multi-neurotransmitter system. J Cytol Histol 2014; 5 4.

[78]   Fu CH, Costafreda SG, Sankar A, *et al.* Multimodal functional and structural neuroimagining investigation of major depressive disorder following treatment with Duloxetine. BMC Psychiatry 2015; 15: 82.

[79]   Ball SG, Atkinson S, Sparks J, *et al.* Long-Term, Open- label, safety study of edivoxetine 12 to 18 mg once daily as adjunctive treatment for patients with major depressive disorder who are partial responder to selective serotonin reuptake inhibitor treatment. J Clin Psychopharmacol 2015; 35: 266-72.

[80]   Rominger A, Cumming P, Brendel M, *et al.* Altered serotonin and dopamine availabilities in the brain of depressed patients upon treatment with escitalopram: a [^{123}I]ß-CIT SPECT study. Eur Neuropsychopharmacol 2015; 25: 873-81.

[81]   Sennfelt, DA, Marques da Silva MA, Tavares AP. Bupropion in the treatment of major depressive disorder in real-life practice. Clin Drug Investig 2011; 31: 19-24.

[82]   McGranahan TM, Patzlaff NE, Grady SR, Heinemann SE, Booker TK. Alpha4beta2 nicotinic acetylcholine receptors on dopaminergic neurons mediate nicotine reward and anxiety relief. J Neurosci 2011; 31: 10891-902.

[83]   Rahman S. Targeting brain nicotinic acetylcholine receptors to treat major depression and comorbid alcohol or nicotine addiction. CNS Neurol Disord Drug Targets 2015; 14: 647-53.

[84]   Luscher B, Fuchs T. GABAergic control of depression-related control brain states. Adv Pharmacol 2015; 73: 97-144.

[85]   Ghose S, Winter MK, McCanson KE, Tammings CA, Enna SJ. The GABAβ receptor as a traget for antidepressant drug action. Br J Pharmacol 2011; 162: 581-90.

[86]   Iodarola ND, Niciu MJ, Richards EM, Vande Voort JL, Ballard ED, Lundin NB, Nugent AC, Machado-Vieira R, Carate CA Jr. Ketamine or other N-methyl-D-aspartate receptor antagonists in the treatment of depression: a perspective review. Ther Adv Chronic Dis 2015; 6: 97-114.

[87]   Pomiemy-Chamiolo L, Poleszak E, Pilc A, Nowak G. NMDA but not AMPA glutaminergic receptors are involved in the antidepressant-like activity of MTEP during the forced swim test in mice. Pharmacol Res 2010; 62: 1186-90.

[88]   Navines R, Martín-Santos R, Gómez-Gil B, Martínez de Osaba MJ, Imaz ML, Castro L. Effects of citalopram treatment on hypothermic and hormonal responses to the 5-HT(1A) receptor agonist buspirone in patients with major depressin and therapeutic response. Psychoendocrinology 2007; 32: 307-12.

[89]   Wang YJ, Yang YT, Li H, Liu PZ, Wang CY, XU ZQ. Plasma galanin is a biomarker for severitiy of major depressive disorder. Int J Psychiatry Med 2014; 48: 109-19.

[90]   Sabban EL, Serova LI, Alaluf LG, Laukova M, Peddu C. Comparative effects of intranasal neuropeptid Y and HS014 in preventing anxiety and depressive-like behavior elicited by single prolonged stress. Behav Brain Res 2014; doi: 10.1016/j.bbr.2014.12.038.

[91]   Keller M, Montgomery S, Ball W, *et al*. Lack of efficacy of the substance P (neurokinin-1 receptor) antagonist aprepitant in the treatment of major depressive disorder. Biol Psychiatry 2006; 59: 216-33.

[92]   Yang LM, Yu L, Jin HJ, Zhao H. Substance P receptor antagonist in lateral habenula improves rat depression-like behavior. Brain Res Bull 2014; 100: 22-8.

[93]   Tsuru J, Ishitobi Y, Ninomiya T, *et al*. The thyrotropin-releasing hormone test may predict recurrence of clinical depression within ten years after discharge. Neuro Endocrinol Lett 2013; 34: 409-17.

CHAPTER 4

Function of Susceptibility Genes

Abstract: The schizoaffective disorder is a heritable disease and some susceptibility genes have been discovered. Risk genes that may encode psychotic symptoms are for example, dysbindin-1 and neuregulin-1 which encode glutamate hypoactivity, catechol-O-methyl transferase and monoamine oxidase A/B which encode dopamine hyperactivity through a decreased dopamine breakdown, and GAD 67 which encodes GABA hypoactivity. The PACAP gene is as well a risk gene for psychotic symptoms. Animals lacking the PACAP gene show behavioral abnormalities which can be ameliorated after administration of 5-HT$_{2A}$ antagonists. The proline hydroxylase is also a risk gene for psychotic symptoms. One haplotype of this gene causes deficits in prepulse inhibition. Rare risk genes for psychotic symptoms may cause a psychosis which begins in the early adolescence and may be treatment-resistant. Environment-gene interactions and epigenetic mechanisms can concern dopaminergic, serotonergic, GABAergic and glutaminergic neurons. Depressive symptoms may be due to alterations of the serotonin and noradrenaline transporter genes. Manic symptoms can be encoded by the genes monoamine oxidase A/B and catechol-O-methyl transferase.

Keywords: Catechol-O-methyl transferase, dysbindin-1, epigenetic mechanism, glutamic acid decarboxylase 67, monoamine oxidase A/B, neuregulin-1, noradrenaline transporter gene, pituitary-adenylate cyclase activating polypeptide, proline hydroxylase, rare genes, serotonin transporter gene, susceptibility gene, treatment-resistant schizoaffective disorder.

4.1. FREQUENT SUSCEPTIBILITY GENES IN SCHIZOPHRENIC SYMPTOMS IN SCHIZOAFFECTIVE DISORDER

Since the development of new methods in genetics and the publication of the human genome, several reports have described the existence of susceptibility genes in schizophrenic and schizoaffective patients. These genes have been identified on chromosomes 8p, 13q and 22q, as well as at other locations in the genome [1]. Here, we shall focus this chapter on 7 frequent genes, namely neuroregulin-1, dysbindin-1, catechol-O-methyltransferase (COMT), monoaminooxidase A/B, proline dehydrogenase, glutamic acid decarboxylase (GAD) 67 and pituitary adenylate cyclase-activating polypeptide (PACAP) [2].

4.1.1. Neuregulin-1: The Glutamate, not the Dopamine?

It has been reported that after haplotype mapping with microsatellites and single nucleotide polymorphisms (SNPs), a neuregulin-1 haplotype appeared as a

Felix-Martin Werner and Rafael Coveñas

susceptibility gene for schizophrenia in patients from Iceland and the United Kingdom [1]. However, the association between the risk gene and schizophrenia is only valid for some haplotypes.

Neuregulin-1 acts as a glial growth factor and also regulates neurotransmitter receptor expression, including the $NMDA2_C$ receptor and the GABA receptor $beta_2$ unit. The expression of the transcripts encoding neuregulin-1 isoforms containing exons 5, 21 or 22 and NMDA receptor-related hybridization have been examined, with the finding that reduced neuregulin-1 subunit transcript expression was restricted to the exon 22-containing isoforms [3]. This observation can be correlated with the glutamate hypoactivity hypothesis in schizophrenia.

4.1.2. Dysbindin-1: The Glutamate, not the Dopamine?

The human dystrobrevin-binding protein 1 locus ($DTNBP_1$), named dysbindin-1, has been shown to be a potential risk gene for schizophrenia [1]. In schizophrenic patients, mRNA dysbindin has been reported in the frontal and temporal cortices, the hippocampus, the thalamus and in other brain regions; reduced levels of mRNA dysbindin were found in the dorsolateral PFC [4]. Reduced dysbindin-1 activities have been reported in the hippocampus of schizophrenic patients [5]. The authors concluded that reduced presynaptic dysbinding-1 activities are frequent in schizophrenia and that they are related to glutaminergic alterations in the hippocampal formation.

Ten DTNBP1 SNPs have been examined in 894 Caucasian individuals, namely 268 patients with a functional psychosis; 483 parents, and 143 siblings. The SNP's found were related the patient's age at onset, the risk for psychosis, and the family neurocognitive background [6]. These authors found different haplotypes of the dysbindin-1 gene; one haplotype (a 5-marker haplotype encompassing exons 2-4) was associated with early-onset psychosis and the other haplotypes were correlated with adult-onset schizophrenia [6]. The authors concluded from their findings that the haplotype of the dysbindin-1 gene was correlated with the form and severity of schizophrenia [6].

4.1.3. Catechol-O-Methyltransferase

The results of both linkage and association studies have suggested that chromosome 22q11 is a locus for schizophrenia. From this gene region, a gene encoding the enzyme catechol-O-methyltransferase (COMT) was identified as a potential candidate for schizophrenia. COMT is an enzyme that catalyses the transfer of a methyl group from S-adenosylmethionine to catecholamines: for example, dopamine (DA).

The SNPs of COMT have been examined and a risk haplotype for schizophrenia associated with a lower expression of the enzyme was found [1]. Since DA breakdown is decreased, increased DA activity is possible. Thus, there is more DA in the synaptic cleft and this can lead to increasing DA activity. This hints at the possible hyperactivity of DA in the mesolimbic system in schizophrenia. Those authors also suggested that the DA D_3 receptor gene and the type 5-HT2$_A$ serotonin receptor gene have a small risk effect [1], although DA and 5-HT hyperactivity have long been assumed to be associated with schizophrenia. Another reason is that atypical neuroleptics, which are very effective in the treatment of schizophrenia, are 5-HT$_{2A}$ and D_2 receptor antagonists and decrease the activities of both DA and 5-HT [7].

4.1.4. Monoamineoxidase A/B

Monoamineoxidases (MAOs) catalyze the metabolism of dopaminergic neurotransmitters [8]. Polymorphisms of the MAOA and MAOB isoforms have been assumed to be susceptibility genes for schizophrenia. Two SNP's, namely rs6323 of MAOA and rs1799836 of MAOB have been assayed in 537 unrelated Chinese schizophrenic patients and 635 healthy controls [8]. The G allele of rs1799836 was identified as a risk factor in the development of schizophrenia [8]. The risk haplotype rs6323T-rs1799836G was found in female schizophrenic patients, but not in male patients. The data confirm MAOB as a susceptibility gene for schizophrenia [8].

4.1.5. Proline Hydrogenase

Proline hydrogenase (PRODH), from the 22q11 region, is a candidate gene for schizophrenia. Six SNPs of PRODH have been found [1]. The authors examined these SNPs in 500 families using the transmission distortion test (TDT). They detected one haplotype of PRODH significantly associated with schizophrenia [1]. In experimental animals, PRODH deficit causes a deficit in prepulse inhibition (PPI) and a sensorineural gating relevant to schizophrenia.

4.1.6. GAD 67

GAD 67 has also been reported to be a susceptibility gene for schizophrenia [9]. It has been described that a decrease in GAD 67 results in low GABA concentrations at the synaptic cleft and a reduction in neurotrophic stimuli.

Using single- and double-label *in situ* hybridization, a decrease in GAD 67 gene expression has been found, and hence reduced concentrations of GABAergic neurons in schizophrenic patients [10]. GABAergic neurons exert an inhibitory effect on projections to the prefrontal cortex (PFC).

It has been reported that a substantial lesion in the mediodorsal thalamus of rats does not decrease mRNA GAD 67 expression in the PFC [11]. Thus, the reduction in the number of neurons in the mediodorsal thalamus is not the cause of a decreased mRNA GAD 67 expression in the PFC.

4.1.7. Pituitary Adenylate Cyclase-Activating Polypeptide

The pituitary adenylate cyclase-activating polypeptide (PACAP) is a risk gene for schizophrenia and schizoaffective disorder [12]. Mice with heterozygous disruption of the PACAP gene show abnormalities in behavior, which can be ameliorated after administration of risperidone, a D_2 and $5\text{-}HT_{2A}$ antagonist, and of ketanserin, a $5\text{-}HT_{2A}$ and $5\text{-}HT_{2C}$ antagonist [12]. PACAP mutant heterozygous mice show deficits in sensorimotor gating after the administration of a $5\text{-}HT_{2A}$ agonist, the hallucinogenic drug $(\pm)$-2,5-dimethoxy-4-iodoamphetamine (DOI) [12].

4.2. RARE SUSCEPTIBILITY GENES AND INCREASED RISK FOR SCHIZOPHRENIC SYMPTOMS: TREATMENT-RESISTANT FORMS OF SCHIZOAFFECTIVE DISORDER

Rare susceptibility genes, which encode neurotransmitter alterations in the brain areas involved in schizophrenic symptoms, can be found in a few patients, but are associated with forms of schizophrenic symptoms that may be treatment-resistant [13]. The first manifestation of schizoaffective psychosis occurs in early adolescence. A rare cause of schizophrenic symptoms combined with extrapyramidal symptoms and loss of consciousness may be due to the synthesis of autoantibodies against the NMDA receptor. This syndrome, which is called anti-NMDA receptor encephalitis, is potentially curable [14]. This autoimmune disease causes glutamate deficiency, and, as a consequence psychotic and extrapyramidal symptoms may occur [14]. A case report of a patient diagnosed with schizophrenia for 7 years who presented an exacerbation of psychotic symptoms with dyskinesia and consciousness disturbances has been described [15]. In the cerebrospinal fluid, autoantibodies against NR1 subunits of NMDA receptors were found, and immunotherapy improved the complaints better than the administration of SGAs. In an exacerbation of psychotic symptoms, anti-

NMDA receptor encephalitis should be excluded by determining autoantibodies against the NMDA receptor [15]. Many of the aforementioned susceptibility genes for schizophrenia are associated with symptoms of bipolar disorder or other psychiatric diseases [13].

4.3. EPIGENETICS IN SCHIZOPHRENIA AND SCHIZOAFFECTIVE DISORDER

Schizoaffective disorder is caused by an interaction of genetic and environmental factors during a period of critical brain development [16]. The relationship between the hypothalamic-pituitary axis and dopamine and serotonin hyperactivity is described in the second and fifth chapters. Epigenetic variations, such as DNA methylation, can involve interactions between any gene and the environment at genome level [16]. Most environmental factors can generate epigenetic mechanisms in schizophrenia and in schizoaffective disorder. Epigenetic mechanisms have been found in the COMT gene, the rheelin gene, and in genes involved in the dopaminergic, serotonergic, GABAergic and glutaminergic pathways [16].

4.4. FREQUENT SUSCEPTIBILITY GENES IN AFFECTIVE SYMPTOMS IN SCHIZOAFFECTIVE DISORDER

4.4.1. Frequent Susceptibility Genes in Depressive Symptoms in Schizoaffective Disorder

In schizodepressive patients, risk genes for schizophrenia are combined with polymorphisms of monoamine transporter genes [17]. 5-HT hypoactivity in the brainstem, mediated *via* 5-HT_{1A} receptors, can be partly due to polymorphisms of the 5-HT transporter gene [17]. In the brainstem, noradrenaline (NA) hypoactivity can be partly caused by polymorphisms of the NA transporter gene [18]. NA hypoactivity is mediated *via* alpha1 noradrenergic receptors.

4.4.2. Frequent Susceptibility Genes in Manic Symptoms in Schizoaffective Disorder

In schizomanic patients, the risk genes for schizophrenia such as COMT, MAO A/B and GAD 67 can elicit schizomanic symptoms. The risk genes COMT and monoamine oxidase A/B encode dopamine hyperactivity in the hippocampus through a reduced breakdown of dopamine. The GAD 67 gene encodes GABA hypoactivity. A reduced presynaptic inhibition of D_2 dopaminergic neurons in the hippocampus can also contribute to dopamine hyperactivity in that region [1]. The

COMT risk gene has been examined in a cohort of schizophrenic and schizoaffective patients and has been correlated with cognitive dysfunction [19]. The authors only found a slight correlation between the risk gene and cognitive deficits [19]. It has been reported that the SLC1A2 gene, which encodes the excitatory amino acid transporter 2 (EAAT2), is found in patients with schizophrenia or bipolar disorder [20]. In rare cases, the SLC1A2 gene has been reported in patients suffering a schizoaffective disorder with a bipolar form [20].

REFERENCES

[1]   Collier DA, Li T. The genetics of schizophrenia: glutamate not dopamine? Eur J Pharmacol 2003; 480: 177-84.
[2]   Harrison PJ, Weinberger DR. Schizophrenia genes, gene expression, and neuropathology: on matter of their consequence. Mol Psychiatry 2004; 10: 40-68.
[3]   Clinton SM, Haroutunian V, Davis KL, Meador-Woodruff JH. Altered transcript expression of NMDA receptor-associated postsynaptic proteins in the thalamus of subjects with schizophrenia. Am J Psychiatry 2003; 160: 1100-9.
[4]   Weickert CS, Straub RE, McClintock BW, et al. Human dysbindin (DTNBP1) gene expression in normal brain and in schizophrenic prefrontal cortex and midbrain. Arch Gen Psychiatry 2004; 61: 544-55.
[5]   Talbot K, Thompson EW, Smith RJ, et al. Dysbindin-1 is reduced in intrinsic, glutaminergic terminals of the hippocampal formation in schizophrenia. J Clin Invest 2004; 133: 1353-63.
[6]   Fatjó-Vilas M, Papiol S, Estrada G, et al. Dysbindin-1 gene contributes differentially to early- and adult-onset forms of functinal psychosis. Am J Med Genet B Neuropsychiatr Genet 2011; 156: 322-33.
[7]   Werner FM, Coveñas R. Classical neurotransmitters and neuropeptides involved in schizophrenia: How to choose the appropriate antipsychotic drug? Curr Drug Ther 2013; 8: 132-43.
[8]   Wei YL, Li CX, Li SB, Liu Y, Hu L. Association study of monoamino oxidase A/B genes and schizophrenia in Han Chinese. Behav Brain Funct 2011; 7: 42.
[9]   Costa E, Grayson DR, Mitchel CP, Tremolizzo I, Veldice M, Guidotti A. GABAergic cortical neuron chromatin as a putative target to treat schizophrenia vulnerability. Crit Rev Neurobiol 2003; 15: 121-42.
[10]   Hashimoto T, Volk DW, Eggan SM, et al. Gene expression deficits in a subclass of GABA neurons in the prefrontal cortex of subjects with schizophrenia. J Neurosci 2003; 23: 6315-26.
[11]   Volk DW, Lewis DA. Effects of a mediodorsal thalamus lesion on prefrontal inhibitory circuitry: implications for schizophrenia. Biol Psychiatry 2003; 53: 285-9.
[12]   Hazama K, Hayata-Takano K, Uetsuki K, et al. Increased behavioral and neuronal responses to a hallucinogenic drug in PACAP heterozygous mutant mice. PLoS One 2014; 9: e89153.
[13]   Haller SC, Padmanabhan JL, Lizano P, Torous J, Keshavan M. Recent advances in understanding schizophrenia. F1000 Prime Reports 2014; 6: 57.
[14]   Werner FM, Coveñas, R. Symptome und therapeutische Möglichkeiten einer Anti- NMDA-Rezeptor-Enzephalitis anhand eines neuronalen Netzwerkes. AMIN 2014; poster 48: 157-158 (www.anim2014.de).
[15]   Huang C, Kang Y, Zhang B, et al. Anti-N-methyl-d-aspartate receptor encephalitis in a patient with a 7-year History of being diagnosed as schizophrenia: complexities in diagnosis and treatment. 2015 Neuropsychiatric Dis Treat; 11: 1437-42.
[16]   Rivollier F, Lotzersztajn L, Chaumette B, Krebs MO, Kebir O. Epigenetics of schizophrenia: a review. Encephale 2014; 40: 380-6.
[17]   Cervilla JA, Molina E, Rivera M, et al. PREDICT study core group. The risk variation at the serotonin transporter 5-HTTLPR genotype: evidence from the Spanish PREDICT Gen cohort. Mol Psychiatry 2007; 12: 748-55.

[18]   Nutt DJ, Demyttenaere K, Janka Z, *et al*. The other face of depression, reduced positive effect: the role of catecholamines in causation and cure. J Psychopharmacol 2007; 21: 461-71.

[19]   Twamley EW, Hua JP, Burton CZ, *et al*. Effects of COMT genotype on cognitive ability and functional capacity in individuals with schizophrenia. Schizophr Res 2014; 159: 114-7.

[20]   Fiorentino A, Sharp SI, McQuillin A. Association of rare variation in the glutamate receptor gene SLC1A2 with susceptibility to bipolar disorder and schizophrenia. Eur J Hum Genet 2014; 23: 1200-6.

CHAPTER 5

Neural Networks in Schizoaffective Disorder

Abstract: In schizophrenic and affective symptoms of the schizoaffective disorder, neural networks are described in the brain regions involved. In schizophrenic symptoms, neural interactions are described in the ventral tegmental area, A10 cell group, hippocampus, prefrontal cortex and hypothalamus. In the hippocampus, the dopamine and serotonin dysfunction is considered. In depressive symptoms, neural networks in the brainstem, including the "mood center" and the center for the circadian rhythm, the hippocampus and the hypothalamus are pointed out. The interaction between the hypothalamic-adrenal axis and the serotonergic system located in the brainstem is included. The involvement of the specific subreceptors of neurotransmitters and neuropeptides, on which prophylactic drugs could exert a therapeutic effect, is discussed.

Keywords: Affective symptoms, brainstem, center of the circadian rhythm, corticotropin-releasing hormone, dopamine, dorsal raphe nucleus, glutamate, hippocampus, hypothalamus, locus coeruleus, medial raphe nucleus, neural network, mesolimbic system, mood center, nicotinic cholinergic receptor, prefrontal cortex, presynaptic inhibition, schizophrenic symptoms, serotonin, ventral tegmental area.

Neural networks have been described in brain areas involved in neurological and psychiatric disease such as major depression, schizophrenia, Alzheimer's disease, Parkinson's disease and generalized epilepsy, and these networks serve as a basis for a multimodal pharmacotherapy with drugs that act at several specific receptors [1-5]. In this chapter, we describe the neural networks in brain areas involved in schizophrenic and affective symptoms in schizoaffective disorder.

5.1. NEURAL NETWORKS IN THE BRAIN AREAS INVOLVED IN SCHIZOPHRENIC SYMPTOMS IN SCHIZOAFFECTIVE DISORDER

In this section, neural networks involved in schizophrenic symptoms in the schizoaffective disorder in the ventral tegmental area (VTA), hippocampus, prefrontal cortex (PFC) and hypothalamus are explored, as seen in Fig. (**1**). These neural networks can be described as follows: in the VTA, tachykinin neurons activate D_2 dopaminergic neurons *via* NK_3 receptors; neuropeptide Y neurons activate D_2 dopaminergic neurons *via* NPY_2 receptors, and gastrin-releasing peptide neurons activate D_2 dopaminergic neurons *via* GRP receptors [6-9]. *Via* Gal1 receptors, galanin neurons inhibit D_2 dopaminergic neurons. Consequently,

Felix-Martin Werner and Rafael Coveñas

NK_3 receptor antagonists, NPY_2 antagonists, GRP receptor antagonists and Gal1 receptor agonists might have an antipsychotic effect. D_2 dopaminergic neurons with high activity, due to the susceptibility genes COMT and monoamine oxidase A/B, transmit a postsynaptic excitatory impulse to glutaminergic neurons [10]. Owing to the dysbindin-1 and neuregulin-1 risk genes, glutaminergic neurons weakly inhibit $5\text{-}HT_{2A}$ serotonergic neurons *via* NMDA receptors. The latter neurons, with high activity, transmit an activating impulse to GABAergic neurons, which owing to the GAD67 gene, weakly inhibit D_2 dopaminergic neurons *via* $GABA_A$ receptors [10]. D_2 dopaminergic neurons activate other D_2 dopaminergic neurons. $5\text{-}HT_{2A}$ serotonergic neurons also activate $5\text{-}HT_{2A}$ serotonergic neurons. In the A10 cell group, D_2 dopaminergic and $5\text{-}HT_{2A}$ serotonergic neurons activate each other and enhance dopamine and serotonin hyperactivity [3].

Via $GABA_A$ receptors, GABAergic neurons located in the VTA weakly inhibit D_1 dopaminergic neurons located in the PFC. D_1 dopaminergic neurons with high activity activate glutaminergic neurons, which weakly inhibit M_4 muscarinic cholinergic neurons *via* NMDA receptors. M_4 muscarinic cholinergic neurons weakly activate GABAergic neurons. Consequently, M_4 receptor agonists could have antipsychotic properties [3]. *Via* NMDA receptors, the glutaminergic neurons in the PFC weakly inhibit $5\text{-}HT_{2A}$ serotonergic neurons located in the VTA. *Via* $GABA_A$ receptors, GABAergic neurons in the VTA inhibit neurotensin neurons located in the PFC, which activate glutaminergic neurons *via* NTS_1 receptors. Consequently, neurotensin analogues and NTS_1 receptor agonists could have an antipsychotic effect [11]. *Via* $GABA_A$ receptors, GABAergic neurons in the VTA inhibit cholecystokinin (CCK) neurons located in the PFC, which weakly activate glutaminergic neurons *via* CCK_A receptors. *Via* CB_1 receptors, cannabinoid neurons strongly inhibit CCK neurons. CCK hypoactivity *via* CCK_A receptors, and cannabinoid hyperactivity *via* CB_1 receptors can induce auditory hallucinations. CCK_A receptor agonists and CB_1 receptor antagonists could be used to treat such hallucinations [12]. Glutaminergic neurons located in the PFC weakly inhibit $5\text{-}HT_{2A}$ serotonergic neurons located in the VTA.

Via $GABA_A$ receptors, GABAergic neurons in the VTA inhibit D_2 dopaminergic neurons located in the hippocampus, which have high activity, and activate glutaminergic neurons. D_4 dopaminergic neurons strongly activate D_2 dopaminergic neurons, and nicotinic cholinergic (nAch) neurons activate D_2 dopaminergic neurons *via* nAch alpha4beta2 receptors. *Via* NMDA receptors,

Brain centers in the schizoaffective disorder (schizophrenic symptoms)

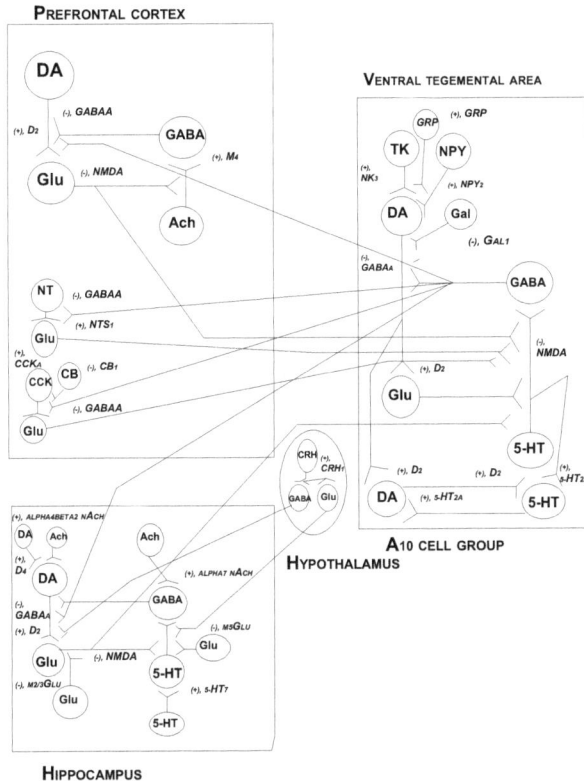

Figure 1: Brain centers in the schizoaffective disorder (schizophrenic symptoms). Neuronal pathways, classical neurotransmitters and neuropeptides involved in schizoaffective disorder (schizophrenic symptoms): 5-HT: serotonin; Ach: acetylcholine; CB: cannabinoid; CCK: cholecystokinin; CRH: corticotropin-releasing hormone; DA: dopamine; GABA: gamma-aminobutyric acid; Gal: Galanin; Glu: glutamate; GRP: gastrin-releasing peptide; NPY: neuropeptide Y; NT: neurotensin; TK: tachykinin; 5-HT$_{2A}$: the 5-HT$_{2A}$ subreceptor of the serotonergic receptor; 5-HT$_7$: the 5-HT$_7$ subreceptor of the serotonergic receptor; alpha4beta2 nAch: the alpha4beta2 nAch receptor of the nicotinic cholinergic subreceptor; alpha7 nAch: the alpha7 nAch subreceptor of the nicotinic cholinergic subreceptor; CB$_1$: the CB$_1$ subreceptor of the cannabinoid receptor; CCK$_A$: the CCK$_A$ subreceptor of the cholecystokinin subreceptor; CRH$_1$: the CRH$_1$ subreceptor of the corticotropin-releasing subreceptor; D$_1$: the D$_1$ subreceptor of the dopaminergic receptor; D$_2$: the D$_2$ subreceptor of the dopaminergic receptor; D$_4$: the D$_4$ subreceptor of the dopaminergic receptor; GABA$_A$: the GABA$_A$ subreceptor of the GABAergic receptor; Gal$_1$: the Gal$_1$ subreceptor of the galanin receptor; GRP: the GRP subreceptor of the gastrin-releasing peptide; m2/3Glu: the m2/3mGlu subreceptor of the metabotropic glutaminergic receptor; m5Glu: the m5Glu subreceptor of the metabotropic glutaminergic receptor; NK$_3$: the NK$_3$ subreceptor of the tachykinin receptor; NMDA: the N-methyl-D-aspartate subreceptor of the ionotropic glutaminergic receptor; NPY$_2$: the NPY$_2$ subreceptor of the neuropeptide Y receptor; NTS$_1$: the NTS$_1$ subreceptor of the neurotensin receptor; A plus mark indicates a postsynaptic excitatory impulse; a minus mark indicates a presynaptic inhibitory impulse.

glutaminergic neurons weakly inhibit 5-HT$_{2A}$ serotonergic neurons and the former neurons are weakly activated by glutaminergic neurons *via* m2/3Glu receptors. 5-HT$_{2A}$ serotonergic neurons with high activity activate GABAergic neurons. 5-HT$_{2A}$ serotonergic neurons are strongly activated by 5-HT$_7$ serotonergic neurons and they are strongly inhibited by glutaminergic neurons *via* m5Glu receptors [13, 14]. Consequently, drugs exerting a 5-HT$_7$ or a m5GluR antagonistic effect could have antipsychotic properties. Nicotinic cholinergic neurons activate GABAergic neurons *via* nAch alpha7 receptors. Glutaminergic neurons in the hippocampus weakly inhibit 5-HT$_{2A}$ serotonergic neurons in the VTA *via* NMDA receptors.

In schizoaffective disorder a relationship has been reported between the hypothalamic-pituitary-adrenocortical axis and dopamine and serotonin hyperactivity [15]. Corticotropin-releasing hormone neurons, located in the hypothalamus, with high activity, transmit an activating impulse *via* CRH$_1$ receptors to GABAergic and glutaminergic neurons. GABAergic neurons, in the hypothalamus, weakly inhibit D$_2$ dopaminergic neurons located in the hippocampus and they can induce D$_2$ dopamine hyperactivity through a reduced presynaptic inhibition if GABA hypoactivity is encoded genetically [15, 16]. Glutaminergic neurons, in the hypothalamus, weakly inhibit 5-HT$_{2A}$ serotonergic neurons *via* m5Glu receptors [15, 16].

5.2. NEURAL NETWORKS IN THE BRAIN AREAS INVOLVED IN AFFECTIVE SYMPTOMS IN SCHIZOAFFECTIVE DISORDER

The neural networks involved in the affective symptoms in schizoaffective disorder in the brainstem, hippocampus and hypothalamus are described (Fig. **2**). They can be described as follows: in the "mood center" of the brainstem, 5-HT$_{1A}$ serotonergic neurons of the dorsal raphe nucleus with a weak activity, due to 5-HT transporter genes, weakly activate GABAergic neurons, which strongly inhibit *via* GABA$_B$ receptors alpha1 noradrenergic neurons located in the locus coeruleus. Alpha1 noradrenergic neurons with a weak activity, due to noradrenaline transporter genes, activate glutaminergic neurons, which strongly inhibit 5-HT$_{1A}$ serotonergic neurons *via* metabotropic glutaminergic (mGlu)5 receptors. Glutaminergic neurons located in the "mood center"of the brainstem inhibit, *via* mGlu5 receptors, other glutaminergic neurons located in the center of the circadian rhythm. Glutaminergic neurons located in the center of the circadian rhythm inhibit, *via* NMDA receptors, 5-HT$_{1A}$ serotonergic neurons of the medial raphe nucleus. The latter neurons activate GABAergic neurons, which *via* GABA$_A$ receptors, inhibit alpha1 noradrenergic neurons located in the locus

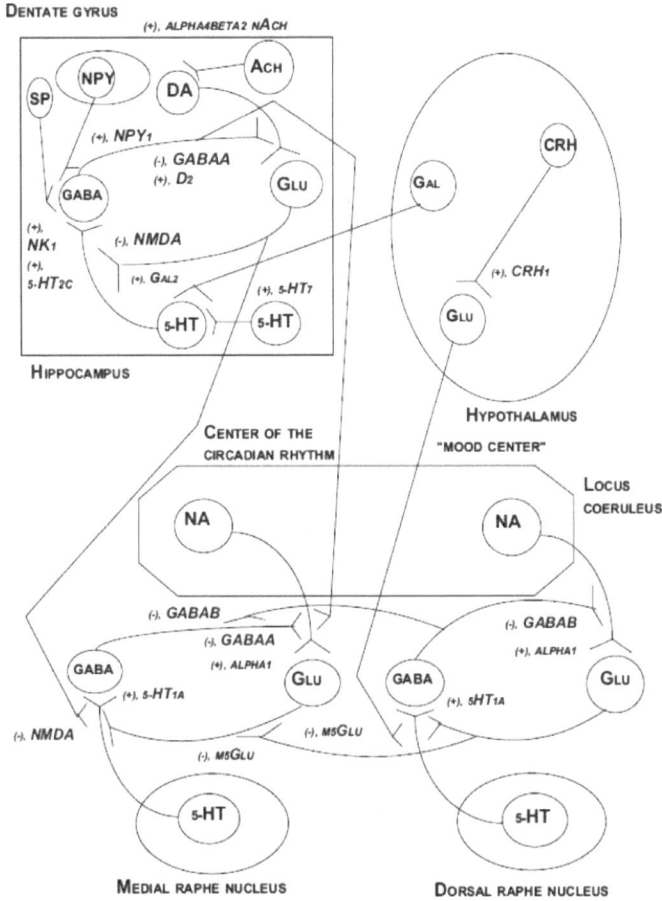

Figure 2: Brain centers in the schizoaffective disorder (affective symptoms). Neuronal pathways, classical neurotransmitters and neuropeptides involved in schizoaffective disorder (affective symptoms): 5-HT: serotonin; Ach: acetylcholine; CRH: corticotropin-releasing hormone; DA: dopamine; GABA: gamma-aminobutyric acid; Gal: Galanin; Glu: glutamate; NPY: neuropeptide Y; SP: substance P; 5-HT$_{1A}$: the 5-HT$_{1A}$ subreceptor of the serotonergic receptor; 5-HT$_{2C}$: the 5-HT$_{2C}$ subreceptor of the serotonergic receptor; 5-HT$_7$: the 5-HT$_7$ subreceptor of the serotonergic receptor; alpha1: the alpha1 subreceptor of the noradrenergic subreceptor; alpha4beta2 nAch: the alpha4beta2 nAch receptor of the nicotinic cholinergic subreceptor; CRH$_1$: the CRH$_1$ subreceptor of the corticotropin-releasing subreceptor; D$_2$: the D$_2$ subreceptor of the dopaminergic receptor; GABA$_A$: the GABA$_A$ subreceptor of the GABAergic receptor; GABA$_B$: the GABA$_B$ subreceptor of the GABAergic receptor; Gal$_2$: the Gal$_2$ subreceptor of the galanin receptor; m5Glu: the m5Glu subreceptor of the metabotropic glutaminergic receptor; NK$_1$: the NK$_1$ subreceptor of the tachykinin receptor; NMDA: the N-methyl-D-aspartate subreceptor of the ionotropic glutaminergic receptor; NPY$_1$: the NPY$_1$ subreceptor of the neuropeptide Y receptor; A plus mark indicates a postsynaptic excitatory impulse; a minus mark indicates a presynaptic inhibitory impulse.

coeruleus. *Via* GABA$_B$ receptors, GABAergic neurons of the brainstem "mood center" inhibit other GABAergic neurons located in the center of the circadian rhythm. Alpha1 neurons activate glutaminergic neurons. In the brainstem center of the circadian rhythm an inverse interaction occurs between alpha1 noradrenergic neurons from the locus coeruleus and 5-HT$_{1A}$ serotonergic neurons from the medial raphe nuclei. Thus, in the medial raphe nuclei, serotonin concentrations are higher during the night and in the locus coeruleus, noradrenaline concentrations are higher during the day. During the course of the day, serotonergic activity decreases, and hence the GABAergic inhibition of noradrenergic neurons also decreases. Consequently, noradrenaline concentrations increase during the day and the glutaminergic inhibition of the serotonergic neurons is also higher. During the further course of the day, noradrenaline concentrations decrease again and serotonin concentrations increase again through reduced presynaptic glutaminergic inhibition [17]. In the hippocampus, D$_2$ dopaminergic neurons with a low activity in depression and a high activity in mania activate glutaminergic neurons which, *via* NMDA receptors, inhibit 5-HT$_{2C}$ serotonergic neurons. *Via* NMDA receptors, glutaminergic neurons located in the hippocampus inhibit 5-HT$_{1A}$ serotonergic neurons located in the brainstem center of the circadian rhythm. In the hippocampus, 5-HT$_{2C}$ serotonergic neurons activate GABAergic neurons, which *via* GABA$_A$ receptors inhibit D$_2$ dopaminergic neurons. *Via* GABA$_A$ receptors, GABAergic neurons inhibit alpha1 noradrenergic neurons located in the brainstem center of the circadian rhythm. Nicotinic cholinergic neurons, *via* nAch alpha4beta2 receptors, activate D$_2$ dopaminergic neurons located in the hippocampus. 5-HT$_7$ serotonergic neurons activate 5-HT$_{2C}$ serotonergic neurons. In the dentate gyrus of the hippocampus, neuropeptide Y neurons activate GABAergic neurons *via* NPY$_1$ neurons, and substance P neurons activate GABAergic neurons *via* NK$_1$ receptors. In the hypothalamus, galanin neurons activate 5-HT$_{2C}$ neurons located in the hippocampus *via* Gal2 receptors. In the hypothalamus, if the hypothalamic pituitary axis is activated, corticotropin-releasing hormone neurons with a high activity transmit a strong activating impulse *via* CRH$_1$ receptors to glutaminergic neurons, which *via* mGlu5 receptors strongly inhibit 5-HT$_{1A}$ serotonergic neurons of the brainstem "mood center" [1, 18].

REFERENCES

[1]   Werner FM, Coveñas R. Classical neurotransmitters and neuropeptides involved in major depression. Int J Neurosci 2010; 120: 455-70.

[2]   Werner FM, Coveñas R. Neuropeptides involved in schizophrenia. Curr Top Neurochem 2005; 4: 35-49.

[3]   Werner FM, Coveñas R. Classical neurotransmitters and neuropeptides involved in schizophrenia: How to choose the appropriate antipsychotic drug? Curr Drug Ther 2013; 8: 132-43.

[4]   Werner FM, Coveñas R. Neuropeptides and classical neurotransmitters involved in Parkinson and Alzheimer diseases. In: Coveñas R, Mangas A, Nárvaez JA, Eds. Focus on neuropeptide research; Trivandrum, Transworld Research Network 2007; pp. 299- 399.

[5]   Werner FM, Coveñas R. Additional pharmacological options in the therapy of generalized epilepsies. Klin Neurol 2010; 41: 37-8.

[6]   Litman RE, Smith MA, Desai DG, Simpson T, Sweitzer D, Kanes SJ. The selective neurokinin 3 antagonist AZD2624 does not improve symptoms or cognition in schizophrenia: a proof-of-principle study. J Clin Psychopharmacol 2014; 34: 199- 204.

[7]   Stadlbauer U, Langhans W, Meyer U. Administration of the Y2 receptor agonist PYY 3-36 in mice induces multiple behavioral changes relevant to schizophrenia. Neuropsychopharmacology 2013; 38: 2446-55.

[8]   Meller CA, Henriques JA, Schwartsmann G, Roesler R. The bombesin/gastrin releasing peptide receptor antagonist RC-3095 blocks apomorphine but not MK-801-induced stereotypy in mice. Peptides 2004; 25: 585-8.

[9]   Ericson E, Ahlenius S. Suggestive evidence for inhibitory effects of galanin on mesolimibic dopaminergic neurotransmission. Brain Res 1999; 822: 200-9.

[10]   Collier DA, Li T. The genetics of schizophrenia: glutamate not dopamine? Eur J Pharmacol 2003; 480: 177-84.

[11]   Kost NV, Meshavkin NV, Batshcheva Elu, Sokolov Olu, Andreeva AL, Miasoedev NF. Neurotensin-like oligopeptides as potential antipsychotics: effect on dopamine system. Eksp Klin Farmakol 2011; 74: 3-6.

[12]   Basoglu C, Oner O, Ates AM, Algul A, Semiz UB, Ebrinc S, Cetin M, Ozcan O, Iipcioglu OM. Association between symptom improvement and change of body mass index, lipid profile, and leptin, grhelin and cholecytokinin levels during 6-week olanzapine treatment in patients with first-episode psychosis. J Clin Psychopharmacol 2010; 30: 636-8.

[13]   Samalin L, Garnier M, Llorca PM. Clinical potential of lurasidone in the management of schizophrenia. Ther Clin Risk Manag 2011; 7: 239-50.

[14]   Vinson PN, Conn PJ. Metabotropic glutamate receptors as therapeutic targets for schizophrenia. Neuropharmacology 2011; 62: 1461-72.

[15]   Haller SC, Padmanabhan JL, Lizano P, Torous J, Keshavan M. Recent advances in understanding schizophrenia. F1000 Prime Reports 2014; 6: 57.

[16]   Ruby E, Polito S, McMahon K, Gorovitz M, Corcoran C, Malaspina D. Pathways associating childhood trauma to the neurobiology of schizophrenia. Front Psychol Behav Sci 2014; 3: 1-17.

[17]   Werner FM, Coveñas R. Klassische Neurotransmitter und Neuropeptide bei der Regulation des Schlaf-Wach-Rhythmus - wie werden neuronale Netzwerke entwickelt? Somnologie 2014; Suppl. 1: 64-65.

[18]   Werner FM, Coveñas R. Classical neurotransmitters and neuropeptides involved in major depression in a multi-neurotransmitter system: focus on antidepressant drugs. Curr Med Chem 2013; 20: 4853-8.

CHAPTER 6

Current Pharmacotherapy in the Treatment of Schizoaffective Disorder

Abstract: The schizoaffective disorder is mainly treated with second-generation antipsychotic drugs as a prophylactic medication. In this sense, the commonly used second-generation antipsychotic drugs are risperidone, olanzapine, quetiapine and aripiprazole. Whereas risperidone has a good antipsychotic, antimanic and therapeutic effect on positive schizophrenic symptoms, olanzapine also exerts a good therapeutic effect on negative schizophrenic symptoms. Quetiapine exerts a good antipsychotic and antidepressant effect. Aripiprazole with a different mechanism of action can improve the outcome of the disease in a long-acting injectable form. Lurasidone is a recently developed antipsychotic drug which can improve cognitive functions as well. Among the mentioned antipsychotic drugs, risperidone causes more often extrapyramidal side effects than the other antipsychotic drugs. When patients suffer from a schizoaffective disorder with a bipolar form, mood-stabilizing drugs can be chosen. Lithium can be administered, because it exerts a secure effect. Other mood-stabilizing drugs are carbamazepine, valproic acid and lamotrigine. Additional pharmacotherapies are sedating neuroleptics, benzodiazepines and anticholinergics or NMDA antagonists to treat the extrapyramidal symptoms. Psychoeducation can improve patient's adherence to the prophylactic medication. At the end of the chapter, the specific subreceptors, on which new drugs could exert an antipsychotic or antidepressant effect, are summarized according to the preceeding chapters.

Keywords: Anticholinergics, aripiprazole, benzodiazepines, carbamazepine, cariprazine, clozapine, lamotrigine, lithium, lurasidone, mood-stabilizing drugs, NMDA antagonists, olanzapine, quetiapine, risperidone, second-generation antipsychotic drugs, sedating neuroleptics, selective serotonin reuptake inhibitors, valproic acid, ziprasidone.

The pharmacotherapy of schizoaffective disorder depends on its form. Schizoaffective bipolar disorder with depressive and manic symptoms should be treated with second-generation antipsychotic and mood-stabilizing drugs [1, 2]. In this chapter, the different mechanisms of action of second-generation antipsychotic (SGA) drugs, their therapeutic effects, and their adverse effects are addressed. The differences between lithium and recently developed mood-stabilizing drugs are also explored [1, 2]. One possibility is the administration of olanzapine as the SGA drug and lithium as the mood-stabilizing drug. In the second case report discussed in chapter 2, the patient suffering from a schizoaffective bipolar disorder was treated with clozapine as a strong SGA drug

Felix-Martin Werner and Rafael Coveñas

and two mood-stabilizing drugs, namely lithium and carbamazepine [3]. A schizodepressive disorder should be treated with SGA drugs combined with mood-stabilizing drugs. As an alternative, selective serotonin reuptake inhibitors could be used. In the case report of the third patient described in chapter 2, who had developed schizomanic psychosis, the disease was treated with a SGA drug, namely olanzapine. It is also recommendable to combine SGA drugs with a mood-stabilizing drug, such as lamotrigine [2]. A new approach in the treatment of schizomanic patients is to administer cariprazine, a new SGA, which has a different mechanism of action and good tolerability and safety [4].

6.1. SECOND-GENERATION ANTIPSYCHOTIC DRUGS

In schizoaffective patients, second-generation antipsychotic drugs (SGAs) are the compounds of choice in the treatment of schizophrenic symptoms [1, 5]. Most SGAs such as risperidone, paliperidone, olanzapine, quetiapine and ziprasidone are combined D_2 and $5-HT_{2A}$ receptor antagonists and they improve positive and negative schizophrenic symptoms. The administration of these SGAs can also be used to treat manic symptoms, because D_2 receptor antagonists improve dopamine hyperactivity in the hippocampus, which is associated with manic symptoms [6]. In the second case report discussed in chapter 2, clozapine, a D_3, D_4 and $5-HT_{2A}$ antagonist and a $5-HT_{1A}$ agonist, was chosen because the auditory hallucinations persisted; these improved after the administration of clozapine [7]. Currently, an injectable application of aripiprazole, a partial D_2 receptor agonist and $5-HT_{2A}$ antagonist, is recommended for the treatment of schizophrenic symptoms [8]. The therapeutic and adverse effects of the recently developed SGAs lurasidone and cariprazine are also addressed below. In the treatment of schizomanic symptoms, cariprazine, a partial agonists at D_2 and D_3 receptors and a $5-HT_{1A}$ agonist, is a promising alternative [4].

6.1.1. Risperidone

Risperidone is a SGA drug with a D_2 and $5-HT_{2A}$ antagonistic effect and it has a higher affinity for the D_2 receptor than olanzapine and quetiapine. Like haloperidol, risperidone improves the score on the Positive and Negative Syndrome Scale (PANSS) and ameliorates negative schizophrenic symptoms better than haloperidol, but to a weaker extent than olanzapine and quetiapine [9]. The weaker therapeutic effect of risperidone on negative schizophrenic symptoms can be explained because risperidone shows weaker affinity for the $5-HT_{2A}$ receptor than olanzapine and quetiapine [10]. The question thus arises of which kind of patients with a schizoaffective disorder could best profit from pharmacotherapy with risperidone. One patient with an obsessive compulsive disorder comorbid with schizoaffective disorder was successfully treated with risperidone at a daily dosage of 4 mg [11]. The administration of quetiapine and risperidone for the treatment of schizodepressive patients was compared in a randomized, open-label, parallel-group study and it was found that quetiapine had a better therapeutic effect than risperidone and that risperidone, in comparison with quetiapine, caused hyperprolactinemia [12]. In 30 psychotic patients, hyperprolactinemia was reported as a result of a monotherapy with risperidone [13]. Aripiprazole, a partial D_2 agonist, $5\text{-}HT_{2A}$ antagonist and $5\text{-}HT_{1A}$ agonist, did not change prolactin levels [5]. Adjunct therapy of aripiprazole was added to the monotherapy with risperidone and normalized prolactin levels were found in 77% of the patients. The authors of that study also found that the psychotic symptoms improved after the administration of risperidone combined with aripiprazole, in comparison with what was observed when monotherapy with risperidone was used [13]. 666 schizophrenic or schizoaffective patients were treated either with long-acting injectable risperidone or with oral quetiapine and the frequency of relapse was explored. Relapse occurred in 16.5% of patients treated with injectable risperidone and in 31.3% of patients treated with oral quetiapine [14]. The authors concluded that injectable risperidone was better able to prevent the relapse of psychosis than orally administered quetiapine [14]. Risperidone has a strong D_2 antagonistic effect and therefore causes extrapyramidal symptoms (EPS). However, it has a lower risk of inducing EPS than first-generation antipsychotic drugs, such as haloperidol, because it undergoes a faster dissociation from the D_2 receptor and also interferes with the $5\text{-}HT_{2A}$ receptor. In sum, it exhibits a higher risk for EPS than olanzapine [1]. Risperidone can cause metabolic and cardiac side effects, such weight gain, hyperlipidemia and increased glucose levels. Risperidone produces weight gain more severely than ziprasidone and aripiprazole, but less severely than olanzapine, quetiapine and clozapine [15]. It can cause hyperlipidemia and increase glucose levels, like quetiapine, but less severely than aripiprazole, olanzapine and clozapine [15]. Because risperidone has a strong D_2 antagonistic effect, it can cause hyperprolactinemia, which can be treated by adjunctive treatment with aripiprazole [13, 16]. Risperidone can cause liver damage, and disturbed liver function was found in 10% of patients treated with risperidone [17]. Neutropenia agranulocytosis are rare side effects observed in antipsychotic treatment with risperidone [18]. Consequently, risperidone is a tolerable and safe SGA for the treatment of schizodepressive and schizomanic psychosis.

6.1.2. Paliperidone

Paliperidone, the active metabolite of risperidone, has the same mechanism of action as risperidone. It is approved for the treatment of schizophrenia and schizoaffective disorder in combination with mood-stabilizing drugs and/or antidepressants [19]. Paliperidone is available as an extended-release form and in long-acting injectable form, paliperidone palmitate [19]. The recommended daily dose of paliperidone is 6 mg/day and this can be increased to 12 mg/day. By increasing the dosage, the therapeutic effect can be augmented, but the dose-related adverse effects can also be increased [19]. Paliperidone improves the PANSS total score, like risperidone, but it exerts a weaker therapeutic effect on negative schizophrenic symptoms than olanzapine [10]. The main route of elimination of paliperidone is *via* renal excretion. Accordingly, paliperidone is recommended instead of risperidone in patients with liver disease [19]. The administration of once-monthly injectable paliperidone palmitate was compared with a placebo in a 15-month study of schizoaffective patients [20]. The authors carried out a prevention trial and compared the costs between the group receiving the once-monthly injectable antipsychotic drug and the control group [20]. The group treated with the long-acting injectable paliperidone had a lower rate of relapse (18.3%) and a lower rate of serious treatment-due adverse effects (3.9%). Consequently, the medical costs for the treatment of schizoaffective patients with the injectable paliperidone were significantly lower than those of a daily oral administration of a SGA [20]. Data about a drug abuser who chronically consumed ketamine, an NMDA antagonist, have been reported [21]. Antagonism at NMDA glutaminergic neurons can induce $5-HT_{2A}$ hyperactivity in the mesolimbic system through a reduced presynaptic inhibition. The patient exhibited agitation and a loss of contact with reality. The psychotic symptoms were very much improved by treatment with paliperidone [21]. Paliperidone can cause EPS to the same extent as risperidone [1]. The cardiac and metabolic side effects of paliperidone are comparable to those caused by risperidone [15]. Since paliperidone has a D_2 antagonistic effect with a high affinity for the D_2 receptor, increased prolactin levels may occur in patients treated with this SGA [16]. Neutropenia and agranulocytosis are rare side effects in the treatment with paliperidone. In sum, paliperidone is a safe and tolerable antipsychotic drug for the treatment of schizodepressive and schizomanic patients. A once-monthly administration of injectable paliperidone palmitate is a safe antipsychotic treatment [20].

6.1.3. Olanzapine

Olanzapine is a SGA with a D_2 and 5-HT_{2A} antagonistic effect. It has a lower affinity for the D_2 receptor and a higher affinity for the 5-HT_{2A} receptor than risperidone [22]. Olanzapine has a stronger antipsychotic effect and improves negative schizophrenic symptoms better than risperidone [9, 10]. This stronger antipsychotic effect is due to the higher affinity for the 5-HT_{2A} receptor [10]. The intramuscular injection of haloperidol combined with lorazepam and of olanzapine in patients with an acute schizophrenia or with schizoaffective disorder, with moderate or severe agitation, has been compared [23]. The authors found that in both groups the PANSS total score decreased in the same way and that agitation was improved in both groups. They concluded that in acute schizophrenia and in acute schizoaffective disorder with agitation the therapeutic effect of the intramuscular administration of haloperidol combined with lorazepam is not lower than that of an intramuscular injection of olanzapine [23]. In an open-label, randomized, controlled study the effects of five antipsychotic drugs - namely haloperidol, amisulpride, olanzapine, quetiapine, and ziprasidone - were explored after treatment of first-episode psychosis in schizophrenia, schizoaffective disorder and schizophreniform disorder [24]. The antipsychotic drugs haloperidol, amisulpride, olanzapine and ziprasidone improved the course of the disease, while quetiapine exerted a lower effect [24]. Olanzapine can cause EPS, but to a lesser extent than risperidone because it has a weaker affinity for the D_2 receptor and a higher affinity for the 5-HT_{2A} receptor [1]. Olanzapine can cause metabolic and cardiac side effects; for example hyperglycemia, hyperlipidemia and weight gain in the same way as clozapine, but more severely than risperidone, paliperidone, quetiapine, aripirazole and ziprasidone [25]. Olanzapine belongs to the prolactin-sparing antipsychotic drugs. Hyperprolactinemia is seldom found in patients treated with olanzapine [16]. The main route of excretion of olanzapine is through the kidney. If kidney function is impaired, the dosage of olanzapine should be reduced [26]. Neutropenia and agranulocytosis seldom occur in patients treated with olanzapine [1]. In sum, olanzapine is a safe and tolerable SGA, with a comparable therapeutic effect to that of other antipsychotic drugs in the treatment of the schizoaffective disorder.

6.1.4. Quetiapine

Quetiapine is a SGA with a D_2 and 5-HT_{2A} antagonistic effect, and a lower affinity for the D_2 receptor and a higher affinity for the 5-HT_{2A} receptor than olanzapine [27]. It rarely causes EPS. Quetiapine is administered in patients with schizophrenia and can be used to treat major depression and generalized anxiety disorders [28]. In a randomized clinical trial of 156 patients with first-episode schizophrenia, the effect of quetiapine at a daily dose of 750 mg and of haloperidol at 14 mg per day on the PANSS total score and the Global Assessment of Functioning (GAF) scale for overall psychosocial functioning was examined [29]. Quetiapine attained significantly better positive and negative scores than haloperidol, but no significant differences were seen in the PANSS total score and the GAF score [29]. The immediate-release and extended-release of quetiapine in Western and Chinese patients with schizophrenia, schizoaffective disorder and bipolar disorder were compared in a pharmacokinetic model. It was found that a twice-daily administration of 200 mg quetiapine or once-daily administration of 300 mg quetiapine in the immediate-release or extended-release form stabilized the course of the disease and afforded good results in the treatment of psychotic and affective symptoms [30]. Quetiapine can be administered to children and adolescents for the treatment of schizophrenia, schizoaffective disorder, and major depression. It is a promising antipsychotic agent because it is a prolactin-sparing drug and seldom causes EPS [31]. However, weight gain and an increased lipid profile should be taken into consideration [31]. Extended-release quetiapine fumarate and risperidone were administered in a randomized, open-label study to patients with schizophrenia and depressive symptoms and patients with schizoaffective disorder and depression [32]. Quetiapine improved the Calgary Depression Scale for Schizophrenia score significantly better than risperidone. Frequent adverse effects following the administration of quetiapine were sedation, somnolence, and dry mouth, and increased prolactin levels were found in 8.1% of the patients treated with quetiapine [32]. As a consequence of the low affinity of quetiapine for the D_2 receptor, the drug causes EPS less frequently than olanzapine. Quetiapine can cause metabolic side effects, *i.e.* weight gain and an increase of glucose and cholesterol levels, to the same extent as risperidone [15]. Quetiapine is a prolactin-sparing antipsychotic drug and only causes raised prolactin levels in 8.1% of patients [32]. Quetiapine is metabolized by the liver and is excreted through the kidneys. In a cases of renal dysfunction, the dosage of quetiapine must be reduced [26].

6.1.5. Ziprasidone

Ziprasidone is a D_2 and $5-HT_{2A}$ antagonist with a preference for the D_2 receptor and shows $5-HT_{1A}$ agonism. It therefore exerts good antipsychotic and antidepressant effects [28]. Like risperidone, ziprasidone decreases the PANSS total score, but has a weaker therapeutic effect against negative schizophrenic symptoms than olanzapine [10]. The antipsychotic effect of ziprasidone was examined in a large cohort of patients with schizoaffective disorder and it was found that switching the antipsychotic to aripiprazole and lurasidone was overlooked by the physicians, although some did consider a switch to risperidone. The authors recommended the application of the long-acting injectable risperidone form [33]. Regarding the Brief Psychiatric Rating Scale (BPRS), switches from other antipsychotic drugs to ziprasidone were explored in a cohort of 67 patients with schizophrenia or schizoaffective disorder at baseline, 4 weeks, 8 weeks, and 12 weeks [34]. The BPRS scale was improved after switching to ziprasidone, but the Clinical Global Impression-Severity (CGI-S) Scale and the GAF Scale were not improved. The body mass index and serum triglyceride levels were significantly improved, but other lipid profiles remained unchanged [34]. 114 subjects with schizophrenia or with a psychotic disorder, switched from other antipsychotic drugs to ziprasidone were explored and metabolic risk factors were measured in a one-year, open-label and prospective study [35]. The authors found that metabolic risk factors such as the body mass index and serum cholesterol levels were considerably improved when the patients were treated with ziprasidone [35]. The adverse effects of ziprasidone can be summarized: ziprasidone can cause EPS, but to a lesser extent than risperidone [27]. This SGA can cause metabolic side effects in 43% of patients [25]. It causes less weight gain and induces a smaller increase in glucose and cholesterol than risperidone, olanzapine and quetiapine [15]. Since ziprasidone is a prolactin-sparing antipsychotic drug, hyperprolactinemia only occurs in a small number of patients [36]. In sum, ziprasidone is a safe and tolerable antipsychotic drug for the treatment of schizophrenia and schizoaffective disorder [1].

6.1.6. Clozapine

Clozapine, which has a D_3, D_4 and $5\text{-}HT_{2A}$ antagonistic effect, has a stronger antipsychotic effect than other SGAs. Clozapine is administered when the psychotic symptoms have not remitted after treatment with other SGAs [27]. Among patients with treatment-resistance, 30% of them responded to treatment with clozapine, another 20% after 3 months, and another 10-20% after 6 months [27]. In a Chinese population, it was reported that clozapine achieved 55.4% decrease of the PANSS total score [7]. Clozapine has a stronger antipsychotic effect because it has a high affinity for the $5\text{-}HT_{2A}$ receptor and because it binds to dopaminergic subreceptors other than the D_2 receptor. D_4 dopaminergic neurons activate D_2 dopaminergic neurons located in the hippocampus. Accordingly, a D_4 antagonistic effect stabilizes hippocampal D_2 dopaminergic neurons. In patients with schizophrenia or schizoaffective disorder, switching from two antipsychotic drugs to single antipsychotic medication was explored and it was observed that switching to a single antipsychotic drug increased the discontinuation rate and that the PANSS total score was lower than when medication was carried out with two antipsychotic drugs [37]. The authors stressed that the treatment with two antipsychotic drugs, and above all the treatment with clozapine, should be maintained [37]. Clozapine deteriorates working performance memory *via* antagonism at the M_1 receptor. However, the major metabolite of clozapine, desmethylclozapine could act as a M_1 agonist. In schizophrenic patients and schizoaffective patients, the serum levels of clozapine and desmyethylclozapine were studied and working performance memory was measured [38]. The authors found that if the clozapine/demethylclozapine ratio decreased, working performance memory was increased. Desmethylclozapine indeed exerts a M_1 agonistic effect. The authors encouraged the administration of cocholinergic agents, for example allosteric modulators of the M_1 receptor, to enhance cognitive functions in schizophrenic and schizoaffective patients [38]. Clozapine is used for the pharmacotherapy of treatment-resistant psychotic disorders and it reduces symptom burden, decreases the risk of suicide, increases the quality of life, and reduces substance use in patients. However, common adverse effects such as constipation, sialorrhea and weight gain, and serious adverse effects such as epilepsy, myocarditis and agranulocytosis, must not be overlooked [39]. Clozapine very seldom causes EPS because in the extrapyramidal system it does not block the D_2 receptor [40]. Clozapine causes metabolic side effects in 45% of patients. It causes weight gain to the same extent as olanzapine and increases glucose and cholesterol levels more severely than risperidone and quetiapine [25]. Because clozapine does not block the D_2 receptor, prolactin levels are not raised [41]. Agranulocytosis and neutropenia occur in 3% of patients treated with clozapine. In order to diagnose neutropenia in these patients, a white cell count should be performed every three weeks [27]. Thus, clozapine should only be chosen to treat treatment-resistant forms of schizophrenia and schizoaffective disorder [27]. If the clozapine dosage is reduced, psychotic symptoms worsen again. Agranulocytosis or neutropenia can be treated by the administration of granulocyte colony-stimulating factors [42].

6.1.7. Aripiprazole

Aripiprazole is an SGA drug with a partial agonism at the D_2 receptor, a 5-HT_{2A} antagonistic effect, and a 5-HT_{1A} agonistic effect, and therefore exerts antipsychotic and antidepressant properties. The antipsychotic effect of aripiprazole has been examined in a meta-analysis and it was reported that the drug elicited a comparable decrease in the PANSS total score to that found for other antipsychotic drugs such as clozapine, quetiapine, risperidone, ziprasidone and olanzapine [43]. In a clinical trial with 59 patients suffering from first-episode schizophrenia, it was found that aripiprazole achieved at least a 20% decrease in the PANSS total score after three weeks [44]. A retrospective study was carried out in which patients were treated with a risperidone long-acting injection or with oral aripiprazole over five years. Among these patients, only 28 of the 84 patients receiving risperidone and only 27 of the 92 patients treated with oral aripiprazole continued with the antipsychotic treatment along the 5-year period [45]. The reasons for discontinuation were lack of effectiveness, adverse effects and/or non-compliance. In some cases, the antipsychotic treatment was switched to treatment with clozapine [45]. In one meta-analysis, the authors examined whether adjunctive treatment with aripiprazole might improve antipsychotic-induced hyperprolactinemia [46]. The proportion of participants who recovered from hyperprolactinemia was found to be significant [46]. Aripiprazole is available as a linker lipid ester, aripiprazole lauroxil, which is injected into the deltoid or gluteal muscle once-monthly. With this administration route (intramuscular), a constant aripiprazole serum level can be achieved. This application of aripiprazole is recommended for the treatment of stable schizophrenia or schizoaffective disorder [47]. The adverse effects of aripiprazole are as follows. Aripiprazole causes EPS less frequently than risperidone because it shows partial agonism at the D_2 receptor [43]. Aripiprazole causes weight gain and increases glucose and cholesterol levels to a lesser extent than olanzapine and risperidone [15]. Aripiprazole is a prolactin-sparing antipsychotic drug and can be used as an adjunctive treatment, for example, with risperidone to normalize prolactin levels [46]. Neutropenia and agranulocytosis are rare adverse effects when aripiprazole is administered [1]. Aripiprazole is a safe and tolerable antipsychotic drug for the treatment of schizoaffective disorder and the once-monthly long-acting injectable application of aripiprazole lauroxil is recommended [47].

6.1.8. Lurasidone

Lurasidone is a recently developed SGA drug with a D_2 and $5-HT_{2A}$ antagonistic effect, a $5-HT_{1A}$ agonistic, and a $5-HT_7$ antagonistic effect. Owing to its mechanism of action lurasidone exerts an antipsychotic and antidepressant effect and improves cognitive function [22]. In a clinical study, 198 out-patients with schizophrenia and schizoaffective disorder were treated with lurasidone. The dosage of the drug was 40, 80 or 120 mg per day. The PANSS total score, and the scores on the Clinical Global Impressions-Severity Scale and the Calgary depression Scale for schizophrenia decreased in all patients as compared to baseline scores. This clinical study demonstrated that lurasidone exerts a good antipsychotic and antidepressant effect [48]. Stable out-patients with schizophrenia or schizoaffective disorder were studied; these patients received

120 mg of lurasidone or 80 mg of ziprasidone once-daily in a double-blind, randomized clinical study lasting 21 days [49]. In both groups, changes in the PANSS total score from the baselines were comparable. The discontinuation rates for lurasidone and ziprasidone were respectively 32.5% and 30.7%. Lurasidone did not cause significant changes in weight, metabolic parameters or in the QT interval in the E.C.G. [49]. The cognitive functions of patients with schizophrenia and schizoaffective disorder treated with 120 mg lurasidone once-daily or with 80 mg ziprasidone once-daily for 21 days were tested [50]. The cognitive functions were gauged using the tests from the MATRICS Consensus Cognitive Battery (MCCB). While ziprasidone had no therapeutic effect on cognitive functions, lurasidone significantly improved them [50]. The adverse effects of lurasidone were as follows. Akathisia was found in 13% of patients and insomnia in 11% of them. Adverse effects such as EPS, hyperprolactinemia, weight gain and increased glucose, cholesterol and triglyceride levels were found to be minor [51]. In brief, lurasidone is safe and tolerable and is a recently developed antipsychotic drug for the treatment of schizoaffective disorder. The drug also improves cognitive functions [50].

6.1.9. Cariprazine

Cariprazine is a new-generation antipsychotic drug showing partial agonism at the D_2 and D_3 receptors with a 10-fold higher affinity for the D_3 receptor than for the D_2 receptor, and it exerts a 5-HT_{1A} agonistic effect [52]. Cariprazine is currently awaiting approval from the US Food and Drug Administration. In schizophrenia, the clinical effect of cariprazine has been explored in comparison to placebo and risperidone at doses of 1.5, 3.0, 4.5, 6.0, and 9.0 mg/day. The decrease in the PANSS total score of cariprazine and of risperidone was higher than that observed in the placebo group, but risperidone showed greater efficacy in the treatment of positive and negative schizophrenia symptoms than cariprazine [52]. The efficacy of cariprazine in the treatment of bipolar mania/mixed episodes and bipolar depression in comparison to placebo was examined in phase II trials. An improvement in the Young Mania Rating Scale (YMRS) total score was achieved in comparison with the placebo after three weeks at doses ranging from 3 to 12 mg per day [52]. The results of treatment of bipolar depression with cariprazine were measured with the Montgomery-Åsberg Depression Rating Scale (MADRS). The depressive symptoms were improved after 8 weeks as compared to the placebo group [52]. Frequent adverse effects in treatment with cariprazine were insomnia, extrapyramidal disorder, sedation, akathisia, nausea, dizziness, vomiting, anxiety, and constipation [53]. No significant changes in metabolic parameters were observed, nor any an increase in prolactin levels, nor a prolongation of the corrected QT interval [53]. Most studies addressing the clinical efficacy of cariprazine have not been published in peer-review journals, but as posters at meetings or as manufactures' press releases [52]. Studies comparing long-term treatment with cariprazine in schizophrenia and in bipolar disorder with other SGA drugs or antimanic drugs are needed in order to evaluate the therapeutic and adverse effects [52].

6.2. MOOD-STABILIZING DRUGS

Mood-stabilizing drugs are administered to patients with schizoaffective disorder, especially if the affective symptoms alternate from depressive to manic symptoms. In some cases, mood-stabilizing drugs are combined with an SGA drug. In case report 1, the SGA clozapine was combined with two mood-stabilizing drugs, namely lithium and carbamazepine [54]. Among the mood-stabilizing drugs, here we describe the mechanisms of action of lithium, carbamazepine, valproic acid, and the newer mood-stabilizing drug lamotrigine [55].

6.2.1. Lithium

Lithium can be administered for the treatment of mania and for the prophylaxis of bipolar disorder or depression. The therapeutic effect in the treatment of major depression is not clear [55]. It would be of great interest to know the real mechanism of action of lithium, since one third of patients treated with lithium have no recurrence of affective symptoms. Lithium decreases the effect of excitatory neurotransmitters such as dopamine and glutamate and increases the inhibitory effect of GABA [55]. It exerts a neuroprotective effect and maintains the volume of the brain regions involved in cognitive functions such as the prefrontal cortex, hippocampus and amygdala. It increases neuroprotective effects mediated through brain-derived neurotrophic factor and B-cell lymphoma 2 and decreases apoptotic processes [55]. The possible adverse effects of lithium are cardio- and nephro-toxicities. This explains why lithium levels should be monitored in treated patients [54].

6.2.2. Carbamazepine

Carbamazepine is an antiepileptic drug and is used as a mood-stabilizing agent. Carbamazepine blocks fast-inactivated sodium channels. According to the literature, it does not exert an agonistic or antagonistic effect on neurotransmitter or neuropeptide receptors [56]. The Bipolar Comprehensive Outcomes Study (BCOS) was a 2-year study carried out on patients with bipolar disorder and schizoaffective disorder and in it the authors compared treatment with conventional mood-stabilizing drugs (CMS) and CMS combined with olanzapine. Relapse rates were similar in both groups. The patients included in this study showed an improvement in their affective symptoms, but remission from the symptoms was not achieved in all patients [57]. In a retrospective study, the additional effect of carbamazepine in the treatment of schizophrenic and schizoaffective patients receiving antipsychotic treatment was investigated [58]. Carbamazepine alone for the treatment of schizophrenic symptoms had no clinical effect and it is only recommended in patients with schizoaffective disorder or in schizophrenic patients with EEG abnormalities [58].

6.2.3. Valproic Acid

Valproic acid is an antiepileptic drug and is used as mood stabilizer in bipolar disorder and in schizoaffective disorder. Valproic acid inhibits GABA channels, enhances the presynaptic inhibitory effect of GABA and stabilizes dopaminergic neurons located in the hippocampus [59]. In one study, forty-eight patients in a manic phase of bipolar disorder with psychotic symptoms, divided into two groups, were examined [60]. The first group received monotherapy with risperidone and the second was treated with risperidone combined with valproic acid. The patients who were only treated with risperidone showed a faster remission of their manic symptoms after three weeks. However, after seven weeks the remission rates were the same in both groups. Patients on monotherapy (risperidone) and those on combined pharmacotherapy developed the same adverse effects [60]. Off-label use of valproate is frequent in psychiatric wards, especially in schizophrenic and schizoaffective patients treated with typical and atypical neuroleptics [61]. The prescription for a mood-stabilizing drug should be calculated very precisely.

6.2.4. Lamotrigine

Lamotrigine is an antiepileptic drug and is used as a mood-stabilizing drug. It blocks voltage-gated sodium channels and alpha4beta2 nAch receptors and hence stabilizes dopaminergic neurons. Additionally, it blocks NMDA receptors and, to a lesser extent, AMPA receptors [62]. Epilepsy is often accompanied by psychiatric comorbidities, such as depression, anxiety disorder, bipolar disorder or psychotic episodes. It has been reported that antiepileptic treatment with lamotrigine can improve psychiatric comorbidity, for example anxiety or psychotic disorders [63]. The administration of mood-stabilizing drugs was studied in 636 hospitalized patients with bipolar disorder, schizoaffective disorder and schizophrenia. The most frequently used mood-stabilizing drugs were lithium, valproic acid and lamotrigine. Over the past few years, the use of these drugs has increased. The affective and psychotic symptoms can be improved, but a longer period of hospitalization is required [64]. Meta-analyses have shown that in clozapine-resistant forms of schizophrenia, adjunctive treatment with lamotrigine has a significant better effect than monotherapy with cloazapine [65].

6.3. ANTIDEPRESSANT DRUGS

Patients with a schizoaffective disorder can show depressive symptoms that can be relieved by treatment with SGA drugs such as quetiapine. If the depressive symptoms are not improved by this treatment, the administration of antidepressant drugs can be attempted [30]. In this case, selective serotonin reuptake inhibitors (SSRIs) or selective serotonin and noradrenaline reuptake inhibitors (sSNRIs) can be prescribed. The noradrenaline and dopamine reuptake inhibitor bupropion is highly effective in the treatment of depressive symptoms, but it can cause psychotic or manic symptoms because it enhances dopamine neurotransmission.

6.3.1. Selective Serotonin Reuptake Inhibitors (SSRIs)

In depressive symptoms in schizoaffective disorder, hypoactivity of brainstem serotonergic neurons occurs; this is mediated *via* the 5-HT$_{1A}$ receptor. SSRIs, for example fluoxetine, paroxetine or citalopram have a therapeutic effect and they can be combined with SGA drugs, which do not interfere with 5-HT$_{1A}$ receptors in the brainstem. Vortioxetine, a recently developed antidepressant drug that modulates 5-HT receptor activity and inhibits the serotonin transporter, was examined at two dosages (10 mg and 15 mg) in patients with major depressive disorder in a randomized, double-blind, placebo-controlled study. After 8 weeks, no significant differences were seen between the control group (placebo) and the groups treated with the two dosages of vortioxetine. Nausea, headache, dry mouth, constipation, diarrhea, vomiting, dizziness, and flatulence were the most frequent adverse effects reported by the patients treated [66]. SSRIs cause adverse effects such as constipation, increased intraocular pressure, ECG abnormalities and sexual dysfunction [67]. Apart from bupropion, mirtazapine and vortioxetine, all SSRIs have the latter side effect. In schizoaffective patients, sexual dysfunction can be due to positive (hallucinations) and negative (anhedonia) symptoms and it may be an adverse effect of most SGA drugs as a consequence of the induced hyperprolactinemia [1].

6.3.2. Other Monamine Reuptake Inhibitors

Since depressive symptoms can also be due to polymorphisms of the noradrenaline transporter gene in the brainstem, it would be possible to administer selective noradrenaline reuptake inhibitors (SNRIs), such as duloxetine and serotonin and noradrenaline reuptake inhibitors (sSNRIs) such as venlafaxine. Antidepressant drugs that enhance noradrenergic neurotransmission can be used to treat the "decreased positive effect", *i.e.* the loss of interest, pleasure and energy. In a 2-year study, the effectiveness of the antidepressant drugs was studied in 150 patients with major depressive disorder and the prevention of the recurrence of depressive episodes was compared. The authors observed that bupropion, a noradrenaline and dopamine reuptake inhibitor that is not appropriate for the treatment of schizoaffective patients, and fluvoxamine, an SSRI, were less effective than other antidepressant drug such as paroxetine, citalopram, both of them SSRIs, duloxetine, an SNRI, and venlafaxine, an sSNRI [68].

6.4. ADDITIONAL PHARMACOTHERAPIES IN SCHIZOAFFECTIVE DISORDER

In patients with schizoaffective disorder, agitation, anxiety, sleep disturbances and EPS can appear as adverse effects after treatment with SGA drugs. If these disturbances are not associated with psychotic symptoms, the following drugs can be administered:

- Sedating neuroleptics such as zuclopenthixol, haloperidol or pipamperon, with a sedating or sleep-inducing effect.

- Benzodiazepines such as lorazepam, which have a sedating/anxiolytic effect.

- M_4 antagonists such as biperiden or NMDA antagonists to treat EPS, although these drugs have a psychotomimetic effect [69].

6.4.1. Sedating Neuroleptics

Agitation, aggression or sleep disturbances may occur in patients with a schizoaffective disorder. These symptoms can appear in an acute episode of psychosis or as a basic symptom. If these symptoms are combined with psychotic symptoms, second-generation antipsychotic symptoms should be combined with a sedating neuroleptic such as pipamperon, levomepromazin or zuclopenthixol. In this context, pipamperon and levomepromazin have a sedating and a weak antipsychotic effect, while zuclopenthixol has an intermediate antipsychotic effect. The above drugs belong to the typical neuroleptics and exert a D_1 and D_2 antagonistic effect [70]. The administration of haloperidol has been explored in psychosis-induced agitation and aggression in comparison to other drugs such as lorazepam, aripiprazole or ziprasidone and it was found that haloperidol exerts a good calming and sleep-inducing effect in these patients [71]. Frequent adverse effects were dystonia and EPS, which in some cases had to be treated with additional anti-Parkinsonian drugs. In some patients, an additional administration of promethazine, a sedating neuroleptic, was necessary [71].

6.4.2. Benzodiazepines

Benzodiazepines have a sedating, anxiolytic, antiepileptic and sleep-inducing effect and exert an agonistic effect at the $GABA_A$ receptor. They can be administered in a psychosis-induced agitation or aggression and, in these cases they can be combined with SGA drugs [72]. The use of benzodiazepines, *e.g.* lorazepam or midazolam, either alone or in combination with antipsychotic drugs, has been examined in patients with psychosis-induced agitation or aggression. When benzodiazepines were administered in combination with antipsychotic drugs, the sedating effect was more marked and the EPS occurred less frequently. However, the administration of benzodiazepines alone was less effective than the use of antipsychotic drugs [72]. The adverse effects of benzodiazepines include sedation, addiction, amnesia, and muscle relaxation.

6.4.3. Treatment of Extrapyramidal Symptoms

EPS, for example akathisia, parkinsonism or dystonia, can be observed as a consequence of treatment with typical neuroleptics and SGA drugs. Typical neuroleptics and the majority of SGA drugs exert a D_2 antagonistic effect. Owing to this therapeutic effect, a neurotransmitter imbalance in the extrapyramidal system with hypoactivity of D_2 dopaminergic neurons and hyperactivity of M_4 muscarinic cholinergic neurons may emerge. In the extrapyramidal system (putamen), M_4 muscarinic cholinergic neurons activate glutaminergic neurons, which inhibit D_2 dopaminergic neurons *via* NMDA receptors. The connection between D_2 dopaminergic and GABAergic neurons is as follows: D_2 dopaminergic neurons located in the caudate nucleus activate GABAergic neurons located in the globus pallidus externus, which weakly inhibit subthalamic glutaminergic neurons *via* $GABA_A$ receptors. The latter neurons activate GABAergic neurons located in the globus pallidus internus, which weakly inhibit M_4 muscarinic cholinergic neurons located in the putamen [73]. Therefore, EPS could also be treated with NMDA antagonists, which enhance dopaminergic neurotransmission through reduced presynaptic inhibition *via* NMDA receptors. The adverse effects of anticholinergics and NMDA antagonists are addressed below.

6.4.3.1. Anticholinergics

Anticholinergics are often administered to treat EPS induced by antipsychotic drugs and because they have a prophylactic effect on these movement disorders. Commonly prescribed anticholinergics are biperiden and trihexyphenidyl. In 20 patients with schizophrenia and schizoaffective disorder, the effect on movement disorders and on cognition was studied after discontinuing the anticholinergic medication [74]. The movement disorders did not worsen and only two cases with remaining akathisia were observed. In these two cases the anticholinergic medication was discontinued, with good results. All twenty patients showed an improvement in cognitive functions after the withdrawal of the anticholinergics. Positive and negative schizophrenic symptoms remained stable after the treatment with anticholinergics had been completed [74]. Anticholinergics can worsen positive schizophrenic symptoms by enhancing dopaminergic neurotransmission through a M4 antagonistic effect [69]. Anticholinergics should only be given if acute EPS occurs. Chronic administration of anticholinergics can enhance the occurrence of tardive dyskinesia [74]. Other adverse effects of anticholinergics are tachycardia, constipation and enlargement of the prostate gland.

6.4.3.2. NMDA Antagonists

In animal experiments, NMDA antagonists, especially antagonists of the NR2B subunit of the NMDA receptor, have been observed to attenuate catalepsy induced by haloperidol, a D_2 antagonist [75]. The authors concluded from their experiments that NMDA receptor antagonists such as amantadine can be used to treat EPS induced by antipsychotic drugs. It should be noted that psychotic symptoms can be induced in animal experiments by the administration of NMDA antagonists and that NMDA antagonists exacerbate schizophrenic symptoms [75]. Accordingly, NMDA antagonists can only be used to treat acute emerging EPS, and only for a short period of time [75].

6.5. NEW PHARMACOLOGICAL OPTIONS IN THE TREATMENT OF SCHIZOPHRENIC SYMPTOMS IN SCHIZOAFFECTIVE DISORDER

In clinical trials, efforts should be made to elucidate whether an add-on therapy using agonists or antagonists of specific subreceptors of classical neurotransmitters and neuropeptides might be able to ameliorate the pharmacotherapy of schizophrenic symptoms in schizoaffective disorder:

- Positive allosteric modulators of the M_4 receptor, which exert an additional antipsychotic effect [76].

- Neurotensin analogues or NTS_1 receptor agonists [77].

- CCK_A receptor agonists to treat chronic auditory hallucinations [78].

- CB_1 receptor antagonists, which increase cholecystokinin levels through a decrease presynaptic inhibition [79].

- Alpha7 nAch agonists, which activate GABAergic neurons in the hippocampus and improve cognitive functions [80].

- 5-HT$_7$ antagonists, which decrease 5-HT$_{2A}$ hyperactivity and improve cognitive functions [81].

- NK_3 receptors antagonists, which decrease D_2 hyperactivity in the mesolimbic system [82].

- NPY_2 receptor antagonists, which decrease D_2 hyperactivity in the mesolimbic sytem [83].

- Antagonists of the gastrin-releasing peptide acting at the GRP receptor [84].

Antipsychotic pharmacotherapy acting at several specific subreceptors of classical neurotransmitters and neuropeptides might improve the therapeutic effect and patients' quality of life.

6.6. NEW PHARMACOLOGICAL OPTIONS IN THE TREATMENT OF AFFECTIVE SYMPTOMS IN SCHIZOAFFECTIVE DISORDER

Clinical trials should be conducted with a view to determining whether the following agonists or antagonists of specific subreceptors of classical neurotransmitters or neuropeptides might improve the treatment of depressive symptoms in schizoaffective disorder.

- $GABA_B$ antagonists, which increase noradrenaline levels through decreased presynaptic inhibition [85].

- m5Glu receptor and NMDA antagonists, which increase serotonin levels [86].

- CRH$_1$ receptor antagonists, which increase serotonin levels through reduced presynaptic inhibition [87].

- GAL2 agonists, which enhance serotonin neurotransmission [88].

- 5-HT$_7$ antagonists.

- NK$_1$ receptors antagonists, which enhance GABAergic neurotransmission [89].

- NPY$_1$ receptor antagonists [90].

A multimodal pharmacotherapy against the affective symptoms in schizoaffective disorder might improve the therapeutic effect of prophylactic medication.

REFERENCES

[1]   Werner FM, Coveñas R. Safety of antipsychotic drugs: focus on therapeutic and adverse effects. Exp Opin Drug Saf 2014; 13: 1031-42.
[2]   Malhi GS, Tanious M, Das P, Coulston CM, Berk M. Potential mechanisms of action of lithium in bipolar disorder: current understanding. CNS Drugs 2013; 27: 135-53.
[3]   Rajina P. Antiepileptic drugs as mood stabilizers: what did we learn from the epileptology? Ideggyogy Sz 2008; 61: 305-16.
[4]   Durgam S, Starace A, Migliore R, Ruth A, Németh G, Laszlovszky I. An evaluation of the safety and efficacy of cariprazine in patients with acute exacerbation of schizophrenia: a phase II, randomized, clinical trial. Schizophr Res. 2014; 152: 450-7.
[5]   Werner FM, Coveñas R. Classical neurotransmitters and neuropeptides involved in schizophrenia: how to improve the therapeutic effect of the antipsychotic drugs. J Pharm Pharmacol 2014; 2: 571-81.
[6]   Bumb JM, Enning F, Leweke FM. Repurposed drugs for the treatment of schizophrenia and bipolar disorder. Curr Top Chem Med 2013; 13: 2364-85.
[7]   Shang DW, Li LJ, Wang XP, *et al.* Population pharmacokinetic/pharmacodynamic model for clozapine for characterising the relationship between accumulated exposure and PANSS scores in patients with schizophrenia. Ther Drug Monit 2013; 36: 378-86.
[8]   Raoufinia A, Baker RA, Eramo A, *et al.* Initiation of aripiprazole once-monthly in patients with schizophrenia. Curr Med Res Opin 2015; 31: 583-92.
[9]   Pilla Reddy V, Kozielska M, Suleiman AA, *et al.* Pharmacokinetic-pharmacodynamic modeling of antipsychotic drugs in patients with schizophrenia Part I: The use of PANSS total score and clinical utility. Schizophr Res 2013; 146: 144-52.
[10]   Pilla Reddy V, Kozielska M, Suleiman AA, *et al.* Pharmacokinetic-pharmacodynamic modeling of antipsychotic drugs in patients with schizophrenia Part II: The use of subscales of the PANSS score. Schizophr Res 2013; 146: 153-61.
[11]   Chiou YJ, Lin PY, Lee Y. Risperidone as monotherapy for a patient with obsessive compulsive disorder comorbid with schizoaffective disorder: a case report. Clin Neuropharmacol 2015; 38: 114-6.
[12]   Kasper S, Montagnani G, Trespi G, De Fiorino M. Treatment of depressive symptoms in patients with schizophrenia: a randomized, open-label, parallel-group, flexible-dose subgroup analysis of patients

treated with extended-release quetiapine fumarate or risperiodone. Int Clin Psychopharmacol 2015; 30: 14-22.

[13]   Ranjbar F, Sadeghi-Bazargani H, Niari Khams P, Arfaie A, Salari A, Farahbakhsh M. Adjunctive treatment with aripiprazole for risperidone-induced hyperprolactinemia. Neuropsychiatr Dis Treat 2015; 11: 549-55.

[14]   Bouillon F, Eriksson L, Burba B, Raboch J, Kaprinis G, Schreiner A. Functional recovery results the risperidone long-acting injectable *versus* quetiapine relapse prevention trial (ConstaTRE). Acta Neuropsychiatr 2013; 25: 297-306.

[15]   Rummel-Kluge C, Komossa K, Schwarz S, *et al*. Head-to-head comparison of metabolic side effects of second generation antipsychotics in the treatment of schizophrenia: a systematic review and meta-analysis. Schizophr Res 2010; 123: 225-33.

[16]   Besnard I, Auclair V, Callery G, *et al*. Antipsychotic- drug-induced-hyperprolactinemia: pathophysiology, clinical features and guidance. Encephale 2013; 40: 86-94.

[17]   Najim H, Islam N. Checking physical care of people on risperidone long term injectable depot. Psychiatr Danub 2013; 25: S171-3.

[18]   Ringbäck Weitoft G, Berglund M, Lindström EA, Nilsson M, Salmi P, Rosén M. Mortality, attempted suicide, rehospitalization and prescription refill for clozapine and other antipsychotics in Sweden-a register-based study. Pharmacoepidemiol Drug Saf 2014; 23: 290-8.

[19]   Citrome L. Oral paliperidone extended-release: chemistry, pharmacodynamics, pharmacokinetics and metabolism, clinical efficacy, safety and tolerability. Expert Opin Drug Metab Toxicol 2012; 8: 873-88.

[20]   Joshi K, Lin J, Lingohr-Smith M, Fu DJ. Estimated medical cost reductions for paliperidone palmitate vs placebo in a randomized, double-blind relapse-prevention trial of patients with schizoaffective disorder. J Med Econ 2015; 22: PMID: 25800457.

[21]   Zuccoli LM, Muscella A, Fucile C, *et al*. Paliperidone for the treatment of ketamine-induced psychosis: a case report. Int J Psychiatry Med 2014; 48: 103-8.

[22]   Tajima K, Fernández H, López-Ibor JJ, Carrasco JL, Díaz-Marsá M. Tratamientos para la esquizofrenia. Revisión crítica sobre la farmacología y mecanismos de acción de los antipsicóticos. Actas Esp Psiquiatr 2009; 37: 330-42.

[23]   Huang CL, Hwang TJ, Chen YH, *et al*. Intramuscular olanzapine *versus* intramuscular haloperidol plus lorazepam for the treatment of acute schizophrenia with agitation: an open-label, randomized, controlled trial. J Formos Med Assoc 2015; 114: 438-45.

[24]   Pijnenborg GH, Timmermann ME, Derks EM, Fleischacker WW, Kahn RS, Aleman A. Differential effects of antipsychotic drugs on insight in the first episode schizophrenia: Date from the European First-Episode Schizophrenia Trial (EUFEST). Eur Neuropsychopharmacol 2015; 25: 808-16.

[25]   Bodén R, Edman G, Reutfors J, Ostenson CG, Osby U. A comparison of cardiovascular risk factors for ten antipsychotic drugs in clinical practice. Neuropsychiatr Dis Treat 2013; 9: 371-7.

[26]   Caccia S. Biotransformation of post-clozapine antipsychotics: pharmacological implications. Clin Pharmacokinet 2000; 38: 393-414.

[27]   Thomas SP, Nandhra HS, Singh SP. Pharmacological treatment of first-eipsode schizophrenia: a review of the literature. Prim Care Companion CNS Disord 2012; 14: PCC.11r01198.

[28]   Maher AR, Theodore G. Summary of the comparative effectiveness review on off-label use of atypical antipsychotics. J Manag Care Pharm 2012; 18: S1-20.

[29]   Amr M, Lakhan SE, Sanhan S, Al-Rhaddad D, Hassan M, Thiabh M, Shams T. Efficacy and tolerability of quetiapine *versus* haloperidol in first-episode schizophrenia: a randomized clinical trial. Int Arch Med 2013; 6: 47.

[30]   Zhou D, Bui KH, Al-Huniti N. Population pharmakokinetic modeling of quetiapine after administration of seroquel and seroquel XR formulations to Western and Chinese patients with schizophrenia, schizoaffective disorder, or bipolar disorder. J Clin Pharmacol 2015; doi: 10.1002/jcph.544.

[31]   Masi G, Milone A, Veltri S, Iuliano R, Pfanner C, Pisano S. Use of quetiapine in children and adolescnets. Paediatr Drugs 2015; 17: 125-40.

[32]   Kasper S, Montagnani G, Trespi G, Di Fiorino M. Treatment of depressive symptoms in patients with schizophrenia: a randomized, open-label, parallel-group, flexible dose subgroup analysis of patients

treated with extended-release quetiapine fumarate or risperidone. Int Clin Psychopharmacol 2015; 30: 14-22.

[33]   Murru A, Hidalgo D, Bernado M, *et al.* Antipsychotic switching in schizoaffective disorder: A systematic review. World J Biol Psychiatry 2015; 9: 1-19.

[34]   Ko YH, Na KS, Kim CE, *et al.* The effectiveness of cross-tapering switching to ziprasidone in patients with schizophrenia or schizoaffective disorder. Psychiatry Investig 2014; 11: 459-66.

[35]   Chue P, Mandel FS, Thierren F. The effect of ziprasidone on metabolic risk factors in subjects with schizophrenia: a 1 year, open-label, prospective study. Curr Med Res Opin 2014; 30: 997-1005.

[36]   Yeon WP, Yooseok K, Yun HL. Antipsychotic-induced sexual dysfunction and its management. World J Mens Health 2012; 30: 153-9.

[37]   Constantine RJ, Andel R, McPherson M, Tandon R. The risks and benefits of switching patients with schizophrenia or schizoaffective disorder from two to one antipsychotic medication: A randomized controlled trial. Schizophr Res 2015; 166: 194-200.

[38]   Rajji TK, Mulsant BH, Davies S, Kalache SM, Tsoutsoulas C, Pollock BG, Remington G. Prediction of working memory performance in schizophrenia by plasma ratio of clozapine to N-desmethylclozapine. Am J Psychiatry 2015; 172: 579-85.

[39]   Lundblad W, Azzam PN, Gopalan P, Ross CA, Pharm D. Medical management of patients on clozapine: a guide for internists. J Hosp Med 2015; 10: 537-43.

[40]   Werner FM, Coveñas R. Possible therapeutic options in Parkinson's disease according to a neuronal network. Neurol Rehabil 2012; 18: 420-1.

[41]   Wang ZM, Xiang YT, An FR, *et al.* Frequency of hyperprolactinemia and its association with demographic and clinical characteristics and antipsychotic medications in psychiatric inpatients in China. Perpect Psychiatric Care 2013; 50: 257-63.

[42]   Khan AA, Harvey J, Sengupta S. Continuing clozapine with granulocyte colony-stimulating factor in patients with neutropenia. Psychopharmacol 2013; 3: 266-71.

[43]   Khanna P, Suo T, Komossa K, *et al.* Aripiprazole *versus* other antipsychotics for schizophrenia. Cochrane Database Syst Rev 2014; 1: CD006569.

[44]   Park YW, Kim Y, Lee JH. Antipsychotic-induced sexual dysfunction and its management. World J Mens Health 2012; 30: 153-9.

[45]   Deslandes PN, Dwivedi M, Sewell RD. Five-year patient outcomes with risperidone long-acting injection or oral aripiprazole. Ther Adv Psychopharmacol 2015; 5: 151-7.

[46]   Meng M, Li W, Zhang S, *et al.* Using aripiprazole to reduce antipsychotic-induced hyperprolactinemia: meta-analysis of currently available randomized controlled trials. Shanghai Arch Psychiatry 2015; 27: 4-17.

[47]   Turncliff R, Hard M, Du Y, Risinger R, Ehrich EW. Relative bioavailability and safety of aripiprazole lauroxil, a novel once-monthly, long-acting injectable atypical antipsychotic, following deltoid and gluteal administration in adult subjects with schizophrenia. Schizophr Res 2014; 159:404-10.

[48]   Citrome L, Weiden PJ, McEvoy JP, *et al.* Effectiveness of lurasidone in schizoprenia or schizoaffective patients switched from other antipsychotic drugs: a 6-month, open-label, extension study. CNS Spectr 2013; 16: 1-10.

[49]   Potkin SG, Ogasa M, Cucchiaro J, Loebel A. Double-blind comparison of the safety and efficacy of lurasidone and ziprasidone in clinically stable out-patients with schizophrenia or schizoaffective disorder. Schizophr Res 2011; 123: 101-7.

[50]   Harvey PD, Ogasa M, Cucchiaro J, Loebel A, Keefe RS. Performance and interview- based assessments of cognitive change in a randomized, double-blind comparison of lurasidone vs. ziprasidone. Schizophr Res 2011; 127: 188-94.

[51]   Stahl SM, Cucchiaro J, Simonelli D, Hsu J, Pikalov A, Loebel A. Effectiveness of lurasidone for patients with schizophrenia following 6 weeks of acute treatment with lurasidone, olanzapine or placebo: a 6-month, open-label, extension study. J Clin Psychiatry 2013; 74: 507-15.

[52]   Caccia S, Invernizzi RW, Nobili A, Pasina L. A new generation of antipsychotics: pharmacology and clinical utility of cariprazine in schizophrenia. Ther Clin Risk Man 2013; 9: 319-28.

[53]   Citrome L. Cariprazine in schizophrenia: clinical efficacy, tolerability, and place in therapy. Adv Ther 2013; 30: 114-26.

[54]   Bumb JM, Enning F, Leweke FM. Repurposed drugs for the treatment of schizophrenia and bipolar disorders. Curr Top Med Chem 2013; 13: 2364-85.

[55]   Malhi GS, Tanious M, Coulston CM, Berk M Potential mechanisms of action of lithium in bipolar disorder: current understanding. CNS Drugs 2013; 27: 135-53.

[56]   Karoly R, Lenkey N, Juhasz AO, Vizi ES, Mike A. Fast- or slow inactivated state preference of Na$^+$ channel inhibitors: a simulation and experimental study. PloS Compact Biol 2010; 6: e10000818.

[57]   Kulkarni J, Filia S, Berk L, Filia K, Dodd S, de Castella A, Brnabic AJ, Lowry AJ, Kelin K, Montgomery W, Fitzgerald PB, Berk M. Treatment and outcomes of an Australian cohort of outpatients with bipolar I or schizoaffective disorder over twenty- four months: implications for clinical practice. BMC Psychiatry 2012; 12: 228.

[58]   Leucht S, Helfer B, Dold M, Kissling W, McGrath J. Carbamazepine for schizophrenia. Cochrane Database Syst Rev 2014; 5: CD001258.

[59]   Kus K, Burda K, Nowakowska E, Czzubak A, Metelska J, Lancucki M, Brodowska K, Nowakowska A. Effect of valproic acid and envinronmental enrichment on behavioral functions in rats. Arzneimittelforschung 2010; 60: 471-8.

[60]   Moosavi SM, Ahmadi M, Monajemi MB. Risperidone *versus* risperidone plus sodium valproate for treatment of bipolar disorder: a randomized, double-blind clinical-trial. Glob J Health Sci 2014; 6: 163-7.

[61]   Horowitz E, Bergmann LC, Ashkenazy C, Moscona-Hurvitz I, Grinvald-Fogel H, Magnezi R. Off-label use of valproate for schizophrenia. PLoS One 2014; 9: e92573.

[62]   Glauser TA, Cnaan A, Shinnar S, *et al.* Childhood absence epilepsy study group. Ethosuximide, valproic acid, and lamotrigine in childhood absence epilepsy. N Engl J Med 2010; 362: 790-9.

[63]   Sepic-Grahovac D, Grahovac T, Ruzic-Barsic A, Ruzic K, Dadic-Hero E. Lamotrigine treatment of a patient affected by epilepsy and anxiety disorder. Psychiatr Danub 2011; 23: 111-3.

[64]   Ventriglio A, Vincenti A, Centorrino F, Talamo A, Fitzmaurice G, Baldessarini RJ. Use of mood stabilizers for hospitalized psychotic and bipolar disorder patients. Int Clin Psychopharmcol 2011; 26: 88-95.

[65]   Tiihonen J, Wahlbeck K, Kivienemi V. The efficacy of lamotrigine in clozapine- resistant schizophrenia: a systematic review and meta-analysis. Schizophr Res 2009; 109: 10-4.

[66]   Mahableshwarkar AR, Jabobsen PL, Serenko M, Chen Y, Trivedi MH. A randomized, double-blind, placebo-controlled study of the efficacy and safety of 2 doses of vortioxetine in adults with major depressive disorder. J Clin Psychiatry 2015; 76: 583-91.

[67]   Waldinger MD. Psychiatric disorders and sexual dysfunction. Handb Clin Neurol 2015; 130: 469-89.

[68]   Buoli M, Cumerlato Melter C, Caldiroli A, Altamura AC. Are antidepressants equally effective in the long-term treatment of major depressive disorder? Hum Psychopharmacol 2015; 30: 21-7.

[69]   Werner FM. Therapiemöglichkeiten medikamentös bedingter extrapyramidal bedingter Störungen. Neurol Int Akt-I 2008; 206 (www.anim2008.de).

[70]   Werner FM, Coveñas R. Neurotransmitter und Neuropeptide bei der Regulation des Schlaf-Wach-Rhythmus – pharmakologische Möglichkeiten, Schlaf zu induzieren. Somnologie 2013; Suppl 1: 66-7.

[71]   Powney MJ, Adams CE, Jones H. Haloperidol for psychosis-induced agitation or agitation (rapid tranquillisation). Cochrane Database Syst Rev 2012; 11: CD009377.

[72]   Gillies D, Sampson S, Beck A, Rathbone J. Benzodiazepines for psychosis-induced aggression or agitation. Cochrane Database Syst Rev 2013; 9: CD003079.

[73]   Werner FM, Coveñas R. Classical neurotransmitters and neuropeptides involved in Parkinson's Disease: a multi-neurotransmitter system. J Cytol Histol 2014; 5: 5.

[74]   Desmarais JE, Beauclair E, Annable L, Bélanger MC, Kolivakis TT, Margolese HC. Effects of discontinuing anticholinergic treatment on movement disorders, cognition and psychopathology in patients with schizophrenia. Ther Adv Psychopharmacol 2014; 4: 257-67.

[75]   Yanahashi S, Hashimoto K, Hattori K, Yuasa S, Iyo M. Role of NMDA receptor subtypes in the induction of catalepsy and increase in Fos protein expression after administration of haloperidol. Brain Res 2004; 1011: 84-93.

[76]   Bubser M, Bridges TM, Dencker D, *et al.* Selective activation of M4 muscarinic acetylcholine receptors reveres MK- 801-induced behavioral impairments and enhances associative learning in rodents. ACS Chem Neurosci 2014; 5: 920-42.

[77]   Oliveros A, Heckman MG, del Pilar Corena-McLeod M, Williams K, Boules M, Richelson E. Sensorimotor gating in NTS1 and NTS2 null mice: effects of d- amphetamine, dizocilpine and NT69L. J Exp Biol 2010; 213: 4232-9.

[78]   Sanjuan J, Toirac I, González JC, Leal C, Molto MD, Nájera C, de Frutos R. A possible association between the CCK-AR gene and persistent auditory hallucinatons in schizophrenia. Eur. Psychiatry 2004; 19: 349-53.

[79]   Eggan SM, Melchitzky DS, Sesack SR, Fish KN, Lewis DA. Relationship of cannabinoid CB1 receptor and cholecystokinin immunoreactivity in monkey dorsolateral prefrontal cortex. Neuroscience 2010; 169: 1652-61.

[80]   Preskorn SH, Gawryl M, Dgetluck N, Palyfreman M, Bauer LO, Hilt DC. Normalizing effect of EVP-6124, an alpha-7 nicotinic partial agonist, on event-related potentials and cognition: a proof of concept, randomized trial in patients with schizophrenia. J Psychiatr Pract 2014; 20: 12-24.

[81]   Samalin L, Garnier M, Llorca PM. Clinical potential of lurasidone in the management of schizophrenia. Ther Clin Risk Manag 2011; 7: 239-50.

[82]   Litman RE, Smith MA, Desai DG, Simpson T, Sweitzer D, Kanes SJ. The selective neurokinin 3 antagonist AZD2624 does not improve symptoms or cognition in schizophrenia: a proof-of-principle study. J Clin Psychopharmacol 2014; 34: 199- 204.

[83]   Stadlbauer U, Langhans W, Meyer U. Administration of the Y2 receptor agonist PYY 3-36 in mice induces multiple behavioral changes relevant to schizophrenia. Neuropsychopharmacology 2013; 38: 2446-55.

[84]   Meller CA, Henriques JA, Schwartsmann G, Roesler R. The bombesin/gastrin releasing peptide receptor antagonist RC-3095 blocks apomorphine but not MK-801-induced stereotypy in mice. Peptides 2004; 25: 585-8.

[85]   Ghose S, Winter MK, McCanson KE, Tammings CA, Enna SJ. The GABAβ receptor as a traget for antidepressant drug action. Br J Pharmacol 2011; 162: 581-590.

[86]   Pomiemy-Chamiolo L, Poleszak E, Pilc A, Nowak G. NMDA but not AMPA glutaminergic receptors are involved in the antidepressant-like activity of MTEP during the forced swim test in mice. Pharmacol Res 2010; 62: 1186-90.

[87]   Nikisch G, Agren H, Eap CB, Czernik A, Baumann P, Mathe AA. Neuropeptide Y and corticotropin-releasing hormone in CSF mark response to antidepressant treatment with citalopram. Neuropsychopharamcology 2005; 8: 403-16.

[88]   Wang YJ, Yang YT, Li H, Liu PZ, Wang CY, Xu ZQ. Plasma galanin is a biomarker for severitiy of major depressive disorder. Int J Psychiatry Med 2014; 48: 109-19.

[89]   Yang LM, Yu L, Jin HJ, Zhao H. Substance P receptor antagonist in lateral habenula improves rat depression-like behavior. Brain Res Bull 2014; 100: 22-8.

[90]   Sabban EL, Serova LI, Alaluf LG, Laukova M, Peddu C. Comparative effects of intranasal neuropeptid Y and HS014 in preventing anxiety and depressive-like behavior elicited by single prolonged stress. Behav Brain Res 2014; doi: 10.1016/j.bbr.2014.12.038.

CHAPTER 7

How to Choose an Appropriate Prophylactic Drug

Abstract: After a schizoaffective disorder is diagnosed, a prophylactic medication is administered in most cases. The second-generation antipsychotic drugs risperidone, olanzapine, quetiapine and aripiprazole are the commonly prescribed drugs in the prophylaxis of psychotic and affective symptoms. Risperidone is an appropriate antipsychotic drug to treat schizophrenic and manic symptoms. Olanzapine has a safe therapeutic effect and the lowest discontinuation rate. Quetiapine can be used to treat schizophrenic and depressive symptoms. The long-acting injectable form of aripiprazole is a prophylactic medication which enhances adherence to the pharmacotherapy. Clozapine is a reserve antipsychotic drug for treatment-resistant psychoses. Under this treatment, a 3 weekly blood cell count should be taken in order to exclude a decreased white cell blood count. It is possible to combine second-generation antipsychotic drugs with each other, for example risperidone and quetiapine. The schizoaffective disorder should be treated with a prophylactic monotherapy, but second-generation antipsychotic drugs could be combined with mood-stabilizing drugs, while lithium is given preferentially in a bipolar form. Psychoeducation and a social integration are of great importance in order to achieve a patients' insight in the disease and to enhance their adherence to the pharmacotherapy.

Keywords: Adherence to the drug, aripiprazole, carbamazepine, clozapine, extrapyramidal symptoms, hyperprolactinemia, lithium, mood-stabilizing drug, olanzapine, psychoeducation, prophylactic medication, quetiapine, risperidone, second-generation antipsychotic drug, social integration, treatment-resistant psychosis, valproic acid.

After a schizoaffective disorder has been diagnosed, prophylactic medication is administered in order to prevent the recurrence of psychotic and affective symptoms. In chapter 2, we referred to three case reports of patients with schizoaffective disorder. In the first case report, the patient developed psychosis with alternating depressive and manic symptoms. Treatment with haloperidol was replaced by a pharmacotherapy regimen with clozapine and two mood-stabilizing drugs, namely lithium and carbamazepine [1]. With this treatment, the patient remained stable and was able to join a self-help group. The patient in the second case report developed psychosis with alternating depressive and manic symptoms. The initial treatment with haloperidol was replaced by clozapine. With the administration of quetiapine, the patient remained stable [2]. The patient is now socially integrated and works part-time as a music teacher. The patient in the third case report, with psychotic and manic symptoms, was initially treated with ziprasidone, but began to have ideations of suicide with this treatment. Currently,

Felix-Martin Werner and Rafael Coveñas

the patient is stable with olanzapine administration [3]. From these case reports, it may be concluded that second-generation antipsychotic drugs are very important in the prophylaxis of schizoaffective disorder and that they can be combined with mood-stabilizing drugs such as lithium, carbamazepine, valproic acid and lamotrigine [4].

7.1. SECOND-GENERATION ANTIPSYCHOTIC DRUGS

To date no methods are available for choosing the appropriate antipsychotic drug for the treatment of schizoaffective disorder [5]. Second-generation antipsychotic drugs are the most appropriate treatment for this disorder. Risperidone, with a greater affinity for the D_2 receptor, can be used to treat schizophrenic and manic symptoms, but it is less effective in the treatment of depressive symptoms [2]. Quetiapine, with a greater affinity for the $5\text{-}HT_{2A}$ receptor, can be chosen to treat schizophrenic and depressive symptoms [6]. There are differences in the adverse effect profiles between risperidone and quetiapine because risperidone causes extrapyramidal symptoms (EPS) and hyperprolactinemia more often than quetiapine [7]. The profile of metabolic side effects between these two second-generation antipsychotic (SGA) drugs is comparable. It would be useful to examine the most frequent susceptibility genes in a large cohort of schizoaffective patients in order to determine which of them can be better treated with antipsychotic drugs showing a greater affinity for the D_2 receptor and which patients can be better treated by antipsychotic drugs showing a greater affinity for the $5\text{-}HT_{2A}$ receptor [5]. Olanzapine is a safe SGA that treats negative schizophrenic symptoms better than other antipsychotic drugs. However, it causes metabolic side effects more often than risperidone and quetiapine [8]. The SGA drug aripirazole exerts antipsychotic and antidepressant effects and can be used for the treatment of schizoaffective disorder [9]. A good long-term effect was achieved with the application of aripiprazole lauroxil as a long-acting injectable form [10]. Clozapine is a SGA drug that can be administered in treatment-resistant forms of schizophrenia and schizoaffective disorder [11]. If patients are treated with clozapine, the blood cell count must be controlled every three weeks in order to diagnose neutropenia or agranulocytosis in the early stages of administration [12]. The therapeutic effect on positive and negative schizophrenic symptoms is higher in comparison with other antipsychotic drugs [11].

Two recently developed SGA drugs are lurasidone and cariprazine; the latter is awaiting approval by the Food and Drug administration [13]. Lurasidone exerts a good antipsychotic and antidepressant effect and improves cognitive functions through a $5\text{-}HT_7$ antagonistic effect [14]. The antipsychotic effect of cariprazine is not as potent as that of risperidone and in acute mania it has a good therapeutic effect [15].

7.2. COMBINATION OF SECOND-GENERATION ANTIPSYCHOTIC DRUGS

In a meta-analysis carried out in Hungary, the authors compared the effectiveness of antipsychotic monotherapy and polypharmacy during long-term treatment of schizophrenia and other psychotic disorders [16]. The SGA drugs commonly used were risperidone, olanzapine, quetiapine and aripiprazole. The discontinuation rate was lower with antipsychotic monotherapy than with the combination of antipsychotic drugs. Whereas the combination of two antipsychotic drugs reduced mortality and the hospitalization rate, antipsychotic monotherapy ensured continuing adherence to the pharmacotherapy more efficiently. The combination of two antipsychotic drugs prevented the recurrence of psychotic symptoms better [16]. In patients with a treatment-resistant form of schizoaffective disorder, a combination of two antipsychotic drugs is not effective. The administration of clozapine, which has a higher therapeutic effect than other SGAs, is preferred [17]. However, the combination of two SGAs with a different receptor-binding profile, *e.g.*, risperidone and quetiapine, or of risperidone and aripiprazole, can treat psychotic symptoms better than monotherapy [17].

7.3. COMBINATION OF SECOND-GENERATION ANTIPSYCHOTIC DRUGS WITH MOOD-STABILIZING DRUGS

Patients with schizophrenic symptoms and a bipolar disorder should be treated with monotherapy, although a combination of antipsychotic drugs with lithium or other mood-stabilizing drugs, *i.e.* lithium or anticonvulsant drugs, is commonly prescribed. Manic symptoms should be treated with mood-stabilizing drugs or antipsychotic drugs. Depressive symptoms should be treated by the SGA quetiapine. Among the prophylactic drugs, lithium should be given preferentially [18]. The effectiveness of antipsychotic drugs in the treatment of schizophrenia and bipolar mania was reviewed [19] and the authors reported that SGA drugs have a good therapeutic and prophylactic effect because they prevent the recurrence of psychotic and manic symptoms and decrease the risk of suicide. Among the SGA drugs, olanzapine is better at preventing the recurrence of psychotic symptoms and has the smallest discontinuation rate [19]. Although a combination of SGA drugs with lithium or other mood-stabilizing drugs is not recommended, this polypharmacy is often administered in schizoaffective patients [18].

7.4. IMPORTANCE OF PSYCHOEDUCATION AND SOCIAL INTEGRATION

Non-adherence to prophylactic medication for schizoaffective disorder is a major problem in outpatients and often leads to a recurrence of their psychotic symptoms and further admission to a psychiatric hospital. Hamann *et al.* [20] interviewed German psychiatrists regarding adherence-enhancing measures for patients with schizophrenia and schizoaffective disorder. They found that patients who had been admitted to a psychiatric hospital as a consequence of non-adherence had seldom received psychoeducation, and they insisted on the importance of psychoeducation for patients and their relatives in order to enhance adherence to the prophylactic medication [20]. Psychoeducation can improve the patients' awareness of the disease and can improve adherence to the prophylactic medication [20]. Moreover, in a long-acting depot form an antipsychotic drug improves the regular intake of the medication and decreases the recurrence of psychotic or affective symptoms [20]. Psychoeducation is very important in the treatment and rehabilitation of psychoses [21]. In the treatment of schizoaffective disorder, psychoeducation can improve patients' awareness of the disease and compliance, *i.e.* adherence to the pharmacotherapy. In talks with the psychiatrist, patients and relatives should be informed about the warning signals of the illness, the stress-vulnerability model, and the importance of regularly taking the prescribed prophylactic drug regularly [21]. Psychoeducation is the most effective psychosocial method to prevent the recurrence of psychotic and affective symptoms [20, 21]. Moreover, social integration is also essential for the prophylaxis of disease symptoms. Therefore, relatives should be included in such psychoeducation sessions.

CONCLUSION

Prophylactic medication for patients with schizoaffective disorder is of great importance. SGA drugs are effective and show a better therapeutic effect than first-generation antipsychotic drugs. The most commonly prescribed SGA drugs are risperidone, olanzapine, quetiapine and aripiprazole. In a long-acting form, the SGA is preferred because compliance is improved and recurrence of the disease symptoms occurs less often. Among these drugs, olanzapine has the lowest non-compliance rate and shows the highest therapeutic effect. A combination of antipsychotic drugs improves the outcome of the disease, but involves reduced compliance. Clozapine is the reserve antipsychotic drug for treatment-resistant forms of schizoaffective disorder. Although the combination of lithium or anticonvulsant drugs with SGAs is not recommended, this combination is administered to many patients with schizoaffective disorder. Non-adherence to the prescribed prophylactic medication is a major problem in psychiatry. Accordingly, the psychoeducation of patients and their relatives is an essential adherence-enhancing measure. Social integration of the patient can at least improve the course of the disease.

REFERENCES

[1]   Constantine RJ, Andel R, McPherson M, Tandon R. The risks and benefits of switching patients with schizophrenia or schizoaffective disorder from two to one antipsychotic medication: a randomized controlled trial. Schizophr Res 2015; 166: 194-200.

[2]   Kasper S, Montagnani G, Trespi G, De Fiorino M. Treatment of depressive symptoms in patients with schizophrenia: a randomized, open-label, parallel-group, flexible-dose subgroup analysis of patients treated with extended-release quetiapine fumarate or risperidone. Int Clin Psychopharmacol 2015; 30: 14-22.

[3]   Huang CL, Hwang TJ, Chen YH, *et al.* Intramuscular olanzapine *versus* intramuscular haloperidol plus lorazepam for the treatment of acute schizophrenia with agitation: an open-label, randomized, controlled trial. J Formos Med Assoc 2015; 114: 438-45.

[4]   Malhi GS, Tanious M, Coulston CM, Berk M Potential mechanisms of action of lithium in bipolar disorder: current understanding. CNS Drugs 2013; 27: 135-53.

[5]   Werner FM, Coveñas R. Classical neurotransmitters and neuropeptides involved in schizophrenia: How to choose the appropriate antipsychotic drug? Curr Drug Ther 2013; 8: 132-43.

[6]   Zhou D, Bui KH, Al-Huniti N. Population pharmakokinetic modeling of quetiapine after administration of seroquel and seroquel XR formulations to Western and Chinese patients with schizophrenia, schizoaffective disorder, or bipolar disorder. J Clin Pharmacol 2015; doi: 10.1002/jcph.544.

[7]   Masi G, Milone A, Veltri S, Iuliano R, Pfanner C, Pisano S. Use of quetiapine in children and adolescnets. Paediatr Drugs 2015; 17: 125-40.

[8]   Bodén R, Edman G, Reutfors J, Ostenson CG, Osby U. A comparison of cardiovascular risk factors for ten antipsychotic drugs in clinical practice. Neuropsychiatr Dis Treat, 2013; 9: 371-77.

[9]   Park YW, Kim Y, Lee JH. Antipsychotic-induced sexual dysfunction and its management. World J Mens Health 2012; 30: 153-9.

[10]   Turncliff R, Hard M, Du Y, Risinger R, Ehrich EW. Relative bioavailability and safety of aripiprazole lauroxil, a novel once-monthly, long-acting injectable atypical antipsychotic, following deltoid and gluteal administration in adult subjects with schizophrenia. Schizophr Res 2014; 159: 404-10.

[11]   Thomas SP, Nandhra HS, Singh SP. Pharmacological treatment of first-eipsode schizophrenia: a review of the literature. Prim Care Companion CNS Disord 2012; 14: PCC.11r01198.

[12]   Lundblad W, Azzam PN, Gopalan P, Ross CA, Pharm D. Medical management of patients on clozapine: a guide for internists. J Hosp Med 2015; 10: 537-43.

[13]   Shonberg J, Herenbrink CK, López L, *et al.* A structure-activity analysis of biased agonism at the dopamine D2 receptor. J Med Chem 2013; 56: 9199-221.

[14]   Citrome L, Weiden PJ, McEvoy JP, *et al.* Effectiveness of lurasidone in schizoprenia or schizoaffective patients switched from other antipsychotic drugs: a 6-month, open- label, extension study. CNS Spectr 2013; 16: 1-10.

[15]   Caccia S, Invernizzi RW, Nobili A, Pasina L. A new generation of antipsychotics: pharmacology and clinical utility of cariprazine in schizophrenia. Ther Clin Risk Man 2013; 9: 319-28.

[16]   Katona L, Czobor P, Bitter I. Real-world effectiveness of antipsychotic monotherapy vs. polypharmacy in schizophrenia: to switch or to combine? A nationwird study in Hungary. Schizophr Res 2014; 152: 264-54.

[17]   Dold M, Leucht S. Pharmacotherapy of treatment-resistant schizophrenia: a clinical perspective. Evid Based Ment Health 2014; 17: 33-7.

[18]   Pfennig A, Bschor T, Falkai P, Bauer M. The diagnosis and treatment of bipolar disorder: recommendations from the current s3 guideline. Dtsch Arztebl Int 2013; 110: 92-100.

[19]   Johnsen E, Kroken RA. Drug treatment developments in schizophrenia and bipolar mania: latest evidence and clinical usefulness. Ther Adv Chronic Dis 2012; 3: 287-300.

[20]   Hamman J, Lipp ML, Christ-Zapp S, Spellmann I, Kissling W. Psychiatrist and patient responses to suspected medication nonadherence in schizophrenia spectrum disorders. Psychiatr Serv 2014; 65: 881-7.

[21]   Kieseppä T, Oksanen J. Psychoeducation in the treatment and rehabilitation of psychoses. Duodecim 2013; 129: 2133-9.

CHAPTER 8

CONCLUSION

Schizoaffective disorder has a prevalance of 0.5% in the general population. Since it elicits complications, above all in acute psychosis (*e.g.*, increased suicidal ideation), premature diagnosis and the administration of treatment according to generally accepted guidelines is of huge importance. Because it has a better prognosis than schizophrenia, correctly prescribed treatment and adherence-increasing measures can improve the outcome of the disease. Moreover, psychoeducation and social integration can help worried patients to accept the disease, to adhere to their treatment, and to be aware of the warning signals of the disease. Schizophrenic symptoms exist at the same time as affective symptoms; for example depressive or manic symptoms as a monopolar form, or alternating depressive and manic symptoms in a bipolar form. If alternating depressive and manic symptoms occur, the recurrence of schizophrenic and affective symptoms may be more frequent than in monopolar forms. In the case reports discussed here, the three patients had different forms and severities of schizoaffective disorder. Consequently, they received different treatments, but all three accepted that they were suffering from the disease and they showed good adherence. The three patients are now socially integrated and have jobs, which gives them some self-satisfaction. The most important susceptibility genes for schizophrenic and affective symptoms were discussed in the chapter 4. Schizoaffective disorder is of course an inheritable disease, but according to the stress-vulnerability model, traumatic events can enhance the occurrence of psychotic and affective symptoms. In the chapter addressing neural networks (chapter 5), the coherence between increased levels of corticotropin-releasing hormone in the hypothalamus and dopamine and serotonin hyperactivitiy in the hippocampus was described. As shown in the chapter looking at the alterations of classical neurotransmitters and neuropeptides, traumatic events can be observed in one third of schizoaffective patients.

These findings suggest that patients worried by the conditions could be helped by appropriate social and family therapy. For schizophrenic symptoms, neural networks in the mesolimbic system, hypothalamus, hippocampus and the prefrontal cortex have been described, as well as in the brainstem, hypothalamus and hippocampus for affective symptoms. The interaction between increased activity of corticotropin-releasing hormone neurons and altered neurotransmitters has been discussed. Moreover, the specific subreceptors on which therapeutic drugs exert their effects are explained. The prognosis of schizoaffective disorder is better than that of schizophrenia, because neurotransmitter alterations tend to return to a balanced state in the mesolimbic system and hippocampus. The most important treatment in schizoaffective disorder is the administration of second-generation antipsychotic drugs, which mostly have an antagonistic effect at D_2 and 5-HT_{2A} receptors. The most commonly prescribed second-generation antipsychotic (SGA) drugs are risperidone, olanzapine, quetiapine and aripiprazole. While risperidone, olanzapine and aripiprazole above all exert a therapeutic effect in schizophrenic and manic symptoms, quetiapine is used to treat schizophrenic and depressive symptoms. Olanzapine has a stronger therapeutic effect, because it has a better therapeutic effect on negative schizophrenic symptoms. It is important to note the SGA clozapine, which can be used for the treatment of treatment-resistant forms of schizoaffective disorder. The long-acting injectable form of SGAs is a form of application that increases patients' compliance and better prevents the recurrence of psychotic and affective symptoms. Among the mood-stabilizing drugs, lithium improves affective symptoms in one third of patients. Other mood-stabilizing drugs are, for example, carbamazepine, valproic acid and lamotrigine, which can be combined with SGAs. According to the neural networks discussed, interaction with the following subreceptors of neurotransmitters or neuropeptides might improve the treatment of schizophrenic symptoms (M_4 receptor agonism, NTS_1 receptor agonism, CCK_A receptor agonism, CB_1 receptor antagonism, 5-HT_7 receptor antagonism, NK_3 receptor antagonism, NPY_2 receptor antagonism and GRP receptor antagonism). The interaction with the following specific subreceptors of neurotransmitters and neuropeptides might improve the treatment of affective, *i.e.* depressive symptoms ($GABA_B$ receptor antagonism, m5GluR antagonism, NMDA receptor antagonism, CRH_1 receptor antagonism, Gal2 receptor agonism, NK_1 receptor antagonism, NPY_1 receptor antagonism).

Here, we have summarized the prophylactic drugs used for the treatment of schizoaffective disorder. However, it is very important to ensure patients' adherence to the pharmacotherapy and to improve their awareness of the disease. In this sense, psychoeducation can improve patients' compliance and their regular consumption of the prophylactic drug. If schizophrenic or affective symptoms reoccur, patients do not tend to adhere to the prescribed pharmacotherapy. Accordingly, social integration, for example in a self-help group and within the family, can help patients and family members to better accept the disease and to follow the prescribed treatment. The choice of the appropriate prophylactic drug and additional sociotherapy and psychoeducation can help to improve the course of the disease and to prevent the recurrence of psychotic and affective symptoms that would require acute treatment.

Subject Index

www.ingramcontent.com/pod-product-compliance
Lightning Source LLC
Chambersburg PA
CBHW041730210326
41598CB00008B/831